Introduction to Clinical Allied Healthcare Workbook

by Debra Garber, RN, BSN, MICN, EMT-P

Clinical Allied Healthcare Series

Kay Cox-Stevens, RN, MA
Series Editor

Career Publishing Inc.
Orange, CA

Series Editor and Executive Director: Kay Cox-Stevens
Editors: Valerie Harris, Jacquelyn Marshall, Laura Mertens
Assistant Editors: Cory Jones, William C. Klein
Illustrators: Alan Borie, Valerie Harris
  Additional Graphics obtained from the LifeART™ Collections from Techpool Studios, Inc., Cleveland, OH.
Production Artists: Valerie Harris, Laura Mertens
Photographs: Page 2-2 courtesy Terry Whitener, Hacienda Heights California. Printed with permission.
  Page 3-2 courtesy K. St. Clair Garber, EMS Options Unlimited, Zephyr Cove, Nevada. Printed with permission.
  Page 20-2 courtesy PhotoDisc, Inc., Seattle, Washinton. Used under license.
Cover Design: Harris Graphics
Cover Photographs: (L) & (R) Courtesy K. St. Clair Garber, EMS Options Unlimited, South Lake Tahoe,
  California. Printed with permission.
  (Center) Courtesy Gazelle Technologies, Inc. Used under license.

This publication is designed to provide accurate and authoritative information in regard to the subject matter covered. It is sold with the understanding that the publisher is not engaged in rendering legal, medical or other professional service. If legal advice or other expert assistance is required, the service of a competent professional person should be sought.

Disclaimer: Information has been obtained by Career Publishing, Inc., from sources believed to be reliable. However, because of the possibility of human or mechanical error by our sources, Career Publishing, Inc., does not guarantee the accuracy, adequacy, or completeness of any information and is not responsible for any errors or omissions or the results obtained from the use of such information. The publisher and editors shall not be held liable in any degree for any loss or injury by any such omission, error, misprinting or ambiguity. If you have questions regarding the content of this publication, the editorial staff is available to provide information and assistance.

ISBN 0-89262-550-3

PRINTED AND BOUND IN THE UNITED STATES OF AMERICA

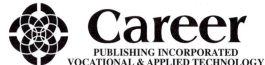

Career
PUBLISHING INCORPORATED
VOCATIONAL & APPLIED TECHNOLOGY
910 N. Main Street,
P.O. Box 5486
Orange, CA 92863-5486

National/Canada
1 (800) 854-4014
Includes Canada, Alaska,
Puerto Rico, and Hawaii

FAX 1-714-532-0180

10 9 8 7 6 5 4 3 2
November 1998

Dedication

This workbook is dedicated to you, the student, a future healthcare worker. Be diligent and disciplined; after all, I may be your patient one day.

Contents

Contents

Welcome to the Student

Thank you for selecting this course of study in the healthcare profession. It is our intent to challenge you to learn, retain the knowledge you acquire, and clinically perform at an excellent level. To help you achieve that goal, this workbook has been created.

This workbook is designed to be used with the *Introduction to Clinical Allied Healthcare Textbook*. It will provide reinforcement of fundamental tools vitally needed within the healthcare profession. As the recipient of those tools and benefits, it is your responsibility to invest time and energy into this course, as well as to complete every exercise contained within the workbook. Allowing the workbook to sit on the shelf will be of no benefit to you, the instructor, or the patient.

As you begin using this workbook, you will notice I have included Study Guidelines. If tests and examinations are difficult for you, this section may provide the *missing link* to successfully completing those parts of the course. After all, every course, career, profession, and vocation involves knowledge, evaluations, examinations, and quizzes.

Use the workbook to its maximum benefit. Review each exercise and then review them again. Work with a study partner and ASK QUESTIONS during class discussion. Remember, healthcare is not a profession in which merely *average* performance is acceptable. You are being educated in order to provide and/or assist with patient care and patient education. Patients depend on each healthcare worker to be competent. Let's not disappoint them.

Have a great time learning!

Debra L. Garber, RN, BSN, MICN, EMT-P
Author

Introduction

To work in the medical field is to make a real contribution to your fellow man. This is a career that will ask much of your mind and heart and give much in return. The satisfaction gained from calming a frightened child or brightening the day of a lonely patient will enrich you. The pride felt will be lasting when your observations and skills someday help to save a patient's life. This is a career where you can really make a difference!

Some of you have already made a decision to seek a career in some area of healthcare. Some of you are just exploring your options. Everything you learn will build a foundation of skills and knowledge, so learn well. Become competent in everything you are taught along the way and be your own taskmaster. We all must be responsible for our own education. If at some point you discover you did not learn a skill well enough, go back and practice until you do. Remember, someday a patient's life may depend on you and your mastery of what you are taught.

Today's healthcare industry places many demands on care givers. We must keep costs down, document everything we do, and have more knowledge and skills than ever before because of new technology. This textbook series was designed to help you build a sound foundation of knowledge and provide many opportunities for cross-training. This workbook is designed to help you learn the skills and information we feel is necessary to build a strong foundation to work in healthcare. The more you can learn, the better. Always remember, however, to practice the art, the science, and the SPIRIT of your new career. Good luck!

Kay Cox-Stevens, RN, MA
Series Editor

Study Guidelines

Throughout the many courses I have instructed within the healthcare profession, one of the most consistent statements I have encountered from students is "I've never been very good at taking tests. I know the material, but I don't do well on tests." Other statements have included "I've always had a personality problem with teachers. They could never explain it to me so that I could understand," and "School is so boring."

I would encourage you not to begin this course with any of those thoughts and feelings. One reason is that you have ELECTED to participate in this course. You must have some interest in the healthcare profession; therefore, the material presented in this course cannot all be boring! To participate means "to have a share; take part; share in an undertaking; the act or fact of taking part." Everyone is partially responsible for making sure they learn the material. So, let's get prepared to give it your absolute best effort and complete dedication.

The following are fundamental keys for achieving success in the classroom, the clinical environment, and during examinations.

1. **Practice your reading skills.** If you recognize a deficiency, discuss it with your instructor. There are many remedial reading programs as well as reading enhancement programs available for today's student. A large part of any course and career includes reading and reading comprehension. Do not be embarrassed or ashamed; take the first step by discussing the possible deficiency with your instructor.

2. **Spell correctly and use proper punctuation.** Basic English skills are important in every area of life; however, you are beginning a career that places great demands on using proper English as well as learning a specialized language (medical terminology). Practice, practice, practice! *Close* is not good enough in the healthcare field. Write, think, and speak the Key Terms and other terms that require reinforcement.

3. **Review basic math concepts.** Healthcare workers must be able to perform basic addition, subtraction, multiplication, and division in their brain and on paper at any time. Calculators may not always be readily available. Your instructor may prohibit their use during various exercises or testing. Be prepared!

4. **Effectively manage your time.** To be of benefit, studying requires a personal investment of time. How much time? To answer that question requires an honest evaluation of your knowledge retention skills, writing skills, memorization ability, reading comprehension, and test-taking skills. Some people read quickly, but have poor retention and comprehension skills. Others may take longer to read an assignment; however, they may possess a near-perfect photographic memory, enhancing knowledge retention. Never be embarrassed to read an assignment and then reread the same material. If that works for you, then do it.

5. **Self-discipline is required if you have a sincere desire to succeed.** Your social life may have to be placed lower on your list of priorities while you develop your study habits for this course.

6. **Decide when understanding the material is more appropriate than memorization.** At first, this may not be obvious; however, attending EVERY class, being attentive during class, and practicing clinical skills will assist you. Repetition from the instructor and/or throughout the textbook is a clue as to what is considered to be important. Complete every exercise, mandatory or optional, for every chapter. These often provide clues as to what is high priority material.

7. **Bring your best classroom manners with you to every class. Be on time, come prepared to take notes, and participate!** It is very distracting to other students and the instructor when students arrive later than expected (emergencies excluded). If you know you are going to be tardy, be courteous and make every effort to notify your instructor. Should you happen to be late, make a quiet entrance and walk BEHIND other students and the instructor to your seat. Do not talk to others as you walk to your seat. Learn how to take lecture notes. Use highlighters or different colored ink pens for emphasis, and cross reference notes (eg, "See page 2.") Actively listen to the instructor to gain clues as to what material may be included on an upcoming examination. Pay attention and DO NOT rely on someone else's notes! For notes to be beneficial, they should be reviewed within twenty-four hours of being written. This will help reinforce the material and perhaps give you an opportunity to identify areas that require clarification from the instructor.

8. **Develop the ability to concentrate; use the skill of active listening.** Sit up straight and do not daydream. Ask questions and participate in activities and discussions. Watching course participants sleep during class is not only distracting, but discouraging to the instructor and other students. Make sure you get enough sleep, eat properly, and limit the ingestion of foods and beverages with poor nutritional value. Some course material may be less intellectually stimulating than other areas; however, it is material that must be learned.

9. **Stay current with classroom work, clinical assignments, special designated work, and skills.** You must make every effort to keep up with the reading assignments. This will be easier if you learn to effectively manage your time. Therefore, if you already know you do not read exceptionally fast, allow more time for those assignments. If you fall behind, it will be very difficult to become current AND learn the material. You will feel left out of classroom discussions and various other activities. Make sure you are current in your skills as clinical time approaches or skill evaluations are being conducted. Falling behind in assignments will greatly reduce your enjoyment of the course, and can be discouraging to both you and the instructor. This often leads to poor test scores, lack of participation, and reduced enthusiasm for the course.

10. **You must understand the requirements of the instructor.** Every instructor has different methods of teaching and may have different requirements. KNOW WHAT THEY ARE! Pay attention to dates of assignments, due dates, examination dates, review dates, skill lab dates, clinical assignments and requirements, group and individual tasks, and when guest lecturers may be presenting. If you have the habit of being tardy, discipline yourself to break it. Patients require procedures on a timely basis; tardiness is inexcusable within the healthcare profession. Ignorance of the instructor's requirements is not an excuse for incomplete work or poor test scores.

Now that the fundamental guidelines have been identified, the following items will relate directly to study time.

1. **Know how to use your textbook as well as the workbook.** Read every page, including the introduction. Thumb through the entire book prior to beginning the course. In other words, get oriented to your book. Look over the various exercises, chapters, the table of contents, and the glossary. Use a highlighter, and frequently review those sections you've highlighted.

2. **Attend every class.** As mentioned previously, it is not wise to be absent, tardy, or lazy with classroom assignments or course participation. It will only hurt you, and possibly your patients.

3. **Prepare a place to study and limit distractions.** Make sure your designated place is free from clutter. Television sets and music should be turned off. Even subtle distractions can reduce the ability to completely concentrate. Let roommates, relatives, and friends know that is your study place. That way, they will know to respect your privacy when you are studying.

4. **Use appropriate study equipment.** DO NOT study on a soft, comfortable sofa, or while lying in bed or sitting on the floor. Have a good, sturdy table or desk with a sturdy chair on which to sit. Sit up straight (this will actually reduce fatigue), and plan to take a break approximately every forty-five minutes. Remember, the brain will only absorb what the buttocks can endure! If you are uncomfortable, sleepy, distracted, hungry, or ill, concentration will be greatly reduced.

5. **Review and recite out loud.** This will assist with reinforcement of the material. Reread your lecture notes, redo the written assignments, review any examinations or quizzes. If extra assignments have been provided, do those also. You can never learn enough in this ever-changing profession.

6. **Talk the new talk.** You will be learning new concepts, terminology, and skills. Talk with your fellow students using the new material. Discuss scenarios, health conditions, and so on. This will also reinforce the new material and assist you with reviewing previously learned information.

7. **Increase retention through the use of mnemonics and association.** Through the use of words or letters, memorization of facts and concepts is often enhanced. Many times this is achieved by listing the first letter of each word and forming another word with those letters that will trigger the facts or concepts. Association involves relating the material to a more familiar area for you.

By implementing the steps provided above, you can prepare for course quizzes and examinations. Here are a few tips and strategies for successful completion of the various course examinations.

1. **Be mentally prepared.** Consistently review and study the course material on a daily basis. *Cramming* the night before the examination usually yields poor results. Make sure you receive a good night's rest prior to the examination. This will allow your brain to function at its maximum potential and actually reduce the amount of stress you may experience.

2. **Be positive.** Coming to the examination prepared will offer the best chances of achieving a high score. Think of the test as a *big homework assignment.* The main purpose of the examination is to evaluate how well you understand the course material. Tests should not be tricky; however, they should force you into using critical thinking skills.

3. **Be properly nourished.** The brain cannot function properly without glucose (blood sugar); therefore, it is important to eat a nutritionally sound meal or snack no later than one hour prior to the exam. If you eat less than 60 minutes before the test, the blood supply is predominantly throughout the digestive system and not the brain. Avoid or reduce the intake of dairy products because chemicals that induce sleep are produced during the digestion and absorption of these foods. You need to be as alert as possible!

4. **Be physically prepared.** Moderate exercise prior to the test has been found to be beneficial by increasing the blood flow to the brain. Blood transports oxygen and glucose—both of which are required for maximum brain function.

5. **Pace yourself.** Manage the time allotted to complete the examination. Wear a watch or know where the clock is in the classroom.

6. **Be properly clothed.** Wear layered clothing so that you can regulate your body temperature in case the temperature of the classroom changes.

7. **Reduce the risk of distractions.** Place yourself away from friends, noises, hallways, and other problem areas.

8. **Pay attention to the answer sheet and the test.** Make sure your answer matches the number of the question on the test. Make sure you have answered all questions. Work problems on a separate piece of paper and make sure your answer is one of the selections provided on the test.

9. **Orient yourself to the exam.** Prior to beginning the examination, skim each page of questions and the choices for answers. Do not panic if you are unsure of the answer to the first question! Proceed until you locate a question you can answer confidently. Just remember to review and check to make sure every question has been answered.

10. **Resist the temptation to change your answers.** Usually, the first answer selected is correct; however, if it is obviously marked incorrectly on the answer sheet, then make the change.

11. **Remember, test taking is a skill.** As with every other skill, it can be learned. Most of the examinations for this course consist of sentence completion, matching, true or false, and occasionally multiple choice or short essay. For sentence completion or short essay questions, you must have some sort of idea as to the information desired. Look for clues to assist you in other areas of the test if possible. True or false questions provide a fifty percent chance of answering correctly. Be careful of terms such as "always" or "never" that may appear within the statement. For multiple choice questions, read and reread the question before selecting an answer. Formulate a response before reading your choice of answers. If your answer is not indicated, determine and eliminate obviously incorrect answers. Usually, multiple choice answers can be narrowed down to two possibilities. Some multiple choice questions may ask you to select the INCORRECT answer regarding the statement. Be very cautious when reading the question.

12. **DO NOT COPY YOUR NEIGHBOR'S ANSWERS!** This is not only dishonest, but your neighbor may have a different examination. Be honest with yourself and your instructor.

Welcome to the healthcare profession! Discipline, dedication, commitment, and a sincere desire to learn are the prerequisites for success in this field. Study hard and study consistently!

Debra L. Garber, RN, BSN, MICN, EMT-P

Contributors

About the Author
Debra L. Garber, RN, BSN, MICN, EMT-P received her Bachelor of Science in Nursing degree from California State University, Bakersfield in 1977. She has 28 years total experience in the Medical and Nursing fields since beginning her career in 1970 by serving as a candy striper. Mrs. Garber has served as a Charge Nurse in various hospital departments including Medical-Surgical, Telemetry, Intensive Care and Coronary Care Units, Pediatrics, Orthopedics, and the Emergency Department. Mrs. Garber is a Mobile Intensive Care Nurse with over 18 years experience. She continues to maintain her Public Health Nurse Certification. In addition, she also performs as an expert witness and a Legal Nurse Consultant.

Mrs. Garber also received recognition as an Outstanding Cardiac Educator from the Central California Heart Institute in 1992 and was nominated as *RN of the Year* in 1993. Currently, Mrs. Garber continues to work as a clinical nurse. She offers her professional services as an allied healthcare education consultant and personal tutor. She also provides clinical preceptorship for students of allied health. In addition, Mrs. Garber has served as Chairperson of the California Rescue and Paramedic Association, CRPA, and is active with the American Heart Association for both Basic Cardiac Life Support and Advanced Cardiac Life Support.

About the Series Editor
Kay Cox-Stevens, RN, MA conceived this textbook series, and recruited and coordinated the authors in the development of each of their texts. She is the author of *Being a Health Unit Coordinator,* and the editor of a Medical-Clerical Textbook Series for Brady. Before entering education, she worked in medical/surgical and critical care nursing and in the inservice department as a clinical instructor.

Formerly a professional development contract consultant for special projects and curriculum development for the California Department of Education, Professor Cox-Stevens has also served as chairperson of the California Health Careers Statewide Advisory Committee, and been a Master Trainer for Health Careers Teacher Training through California Polytechnic University of Pomona. She also is a founding member of the national association of Health Unit Coordinators. Professor Cox-Stevens is currently Program Coordinator of the Medical Assistant Program at Saddleback College in Mission Viejo, California, and operates her consulting business, Achiever's Development Enterprises.

Editor's Note

I would like to take this opportunity to thank Debra Garber for her outstanding work on this book. Through her efforts, she has made this Workbook an excellent and readable educational tool.

I would also like to express my sincere gratitude to the staff of Career Publishing, Inc. and most particularly to Valerie Harris, Senior Editor and Project Coordinator, and Laura Mertens and Jacquelyn Marshall for their editorial contributions. I also would like to express my appreciation to Harold Haase, Publisher, for his enthusiasm for this project and for his humanistic approach to education.

Kay Cox-Stevens, RN, MA
Series Editor

Chapter One
Introduction to Healthcare Facilities

Objectives

After completing this chapter you should be able to
do the following:

1. Define and correctly spell each of the key terms.

2. Name the most important aspect of quality patient care.

3. Briefly describe the historical perspective of
   healthcare facilities.

4. Identify at least two current trends in modern healthcare.

5. Describe at least three services offered by nonprofit
   organizations.

Key Terms

- acute
- asepsis
- chronic

- contagious
- hospitalis
- nonprofit agency

Chapter Overview

Chapter One of the *Introduction to Clinical Allied Healthcare* textbook is devoted to discussing the history of healthcare facilities, as well as the various types of facilities that have evolved over the years. The chapter also provides a brief introduction to health insurance plans and nonprofit organizations.

Because there are so many different types of healthcare facilities, today's healthcare workers have a lot of options available to them. This instructional course will provide you with information and skills that will be useful in a variety of the healthcare settings. Hospitals value workers who have multiple skills (cross-training), so continue to learn new things whenever you can—and explore your options!

Reading Assignment

Read pages 1-1 through 1-7.

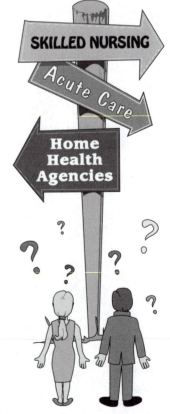

Explore your options!

Name _____

Date _____

Student Enrichment Activities

Complete the following statements.

1. The term *hospital* is derived from the Latin word, _____, which means an institution for guests.

2. During the _____, most hospitals were dark, overcrowded, and dirty.

3. _____ is a condition in which no pathogen, infection, or any form of life is present.

4. X-rays were introduced in the late _____.

5. The _____ _____ is the most important aspect of quality patient care.

6. The _____ _____ _____ are hospitals that provide short-term healthcare to patients.

7. An extended care facility in which skilled nursing services are available at all times is called a _____ _____ _____.

8. Patients with a slow-progressing illness are often cared for in a _____ _____ _____.

9. _____ _____ _____ provide non-emergency care.

10. A prepaid healthcare plan that is directed toward healthcare prevention is called a _____ _____ _____.

11. Organizations that are supported only through contributions are

_____ _____.

Unscramble the following terms.

12. TALHSIOPSI   _____

13. LICIYATF   _____

14. EMNATL TEHLAH   _____ _____

15. EIDCLMA FOFCEI   _____ _____

16. TRNOINPFO   _____

17. GRUINNS   _____

18. TRENGU   _____

19. ITEANNAMECN   _____

20. MUTYNOMIC   _____

21. TRAINONAZOIG   _____

22. PASSESI   _____

23. NYCAGE   _____

24. LKESILD USIGRNN   _____ _____

Name _____

Date _____

Additional Enrichment Activities

Circle the correct answer.

25. The term *hospitalis* means:

    A. a place for sick and injured people.

    B. a place to provide entertainment.

    C. a house or institution for guests.

    D. hospital.

26. An example of a Health Maintenance Organization (HMO) is:

    A. the American Heart Association.

    B. Cardiac Rehabilitation Center.

    C. a health fitness center.

    D. Secure Horizons.

27. Each of the following is an example of a nonprofit organization EXCEPT:

    A. the American Heart Association.

    B. a Health Maintenance Organization.

    C. Mothers Against Drunk Drivers.

    D. the American Cancer Society.

28. The most important aspect of quality patient care is:

    A. asepsis.

    B. the healthcare worker.

    C. research and public education.

    D. the doctor's decisions.

29. "Sudden onset; short duration" describes:

    A. acute illnesses.

    B. payment reimbursement for healthcare services.

    C. chronic illnesses.

    D. asepsis.

Complete the following exercises.

30. Briefly describe the history of healthcare facilities.

    _____

    _____

    _____

    _____

    _____

    _____

    _____

31. List three types of extended or long-term care facilities and describe the type of patient that may receive care in each one.

    _____

    _____

    _____

    _____

    _____

    _____

32. Name and describe two types of community healthcare facilities.

    _____

    _____

    _____

    _____

Name _____

Date _____

33. List at least three types of patient services provided by an urgent care center.

_____

_____

_____

_____

34. Identify at least four examples of nonprofit organizations.

_____

_____

_____

_____

_____

_____

Name _____

Date _____

Introduction to Healthcare Facilities—Puzzle 1

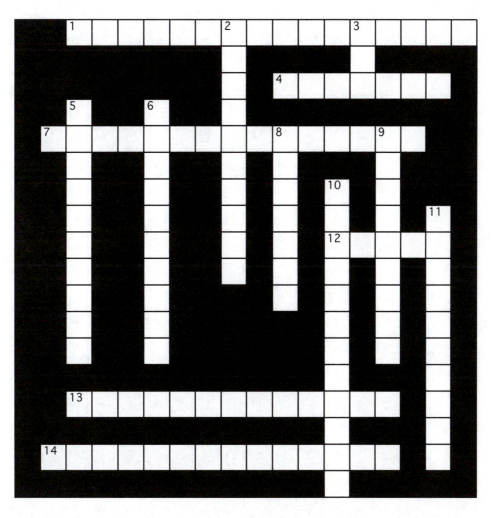

Across

1. _____ _____ facilities provide care to people experiencing emotional and psychological dysfunction (2 words)
4. Slow to develop, persisting for a long time
7. An organization that is supported only by contributions (2 words)
12. Sudden onset, short duration
13. A facility where a physician provides a wide variety of services to patients, but not overnight healthcare (2 words)
14. A type of extended care facility that has nurses available to provide various services (2 words)

Down

2. Latin for "institution for guests"
3. Health maintenance organization
5. Extended healthcare in the home (2 words)
6. A walk-in, free-standing non-emergency care clinic (2 words)
8. A condition in which no pathogen, infection, or any form of life is present
9. A facility that provides care to the general public; with 11 Down
10. A healthcare facility that is usually formed by several doctors who share a common building (2 words)
11. See 9 Down

Name _____

Date _____

Introduction to Healthcare Facilities—Puzzle 2

Find the listed words in the puzzle and circle them. (Contains backwards words.)

S	A	C	Y	D	X	E	R	A	C	H	T	L	A	E	H	C	S
K	T	C	H	C	E	R	A	C	T	N	E	G	R	U	O	I	C
I	S	H	U	R	N	B	U	V	D	U	R	Q	T	M	S	L	O
L	M	O	O	T	O	E	U	P	J	C	S	E	M	P	I	S	U
L	E	S	H	L	E	N	G	R	L	B	N	U	E	N	X	M	T
E	R	P	J	K	T	E	I	A	H	N	N	S	I	N	Q	W	P
D	A	I	M	U	T	W	O	C	T	I	A	C	K	X	O	V	A
N	C	T	U	E	S	T	B	Y	T	I	S	U	O	J	R	O	T
U	D	A	U	Q	W	P	M	Y	S	L	F	S	D	I	S	O	I
R	E	L	P	I	W	X	H	U	V	S	A	O	Q	N	B	F	E
S	D	I	C	K	E	E	O	K	X	N	D	T	R	Z	Y	U	N
I	N	S	B	I	A	I	P	F	Y	P	X	X	I	P	Y	J	T
N	E	C	V	L	G	Z	V	B	B	O	K	V	G	P	N	G	K
G	T	D	T	A	T	W	Z	U	C	F	D	U	D	J	S	O	M
K	X	H	T	E	I	F	Z	P	D	J	C	W	Z	H	O	O	N
L	E	N	R	S	V	H	T	L	A	E	H	E	M	O	H	M	H
A	O	A	O	A	H	T	L	A	E	H	L	A	T	N	E	M	H
C	C	M	E	D	I	C	A	L	O	F	F	I	C	E	C	O	J

ACUTE	EXTENDED CARE	MENTAL HEALTH
ASEPSIS	HEALTHCARE	NONPROFIT AGENCY
CARE	HMO	OUTPATIENT
CHRONIC	HOME HEALTH	SKILLED NURSING
CLINICS	HOSPITAL	URGENT CARE
COMMUNITY HEALTH	HOSPITALIS	
CONTAGIOUS	MEDICAL OFFICE	

Chapter Two
The Acute Care Hospital

Objectives

After completing this chapter you should be able to
do the following:

1. Define and correctly spell each of the key terms.

2. Explain the purpose of the organizational structure of a
    healthcare facility.

3. List and describe the main function of at least five types
    of acute care hospitals.

4. Briefly explain the main functions of four general
    classifications of hospital departments.

5. Identify at least six branches of Nursing Services and
    describe the type of care they provide.

6. Name two of the most serious infections to which
    healthcare workers may be exposed.

Key Terms

- chain of command
- critical care
- myocardial infarction

- rooming-in
- sterilization
- wellness

Chapter Overview

Chapter Two of the textbook serves three purposes. The first is to acquaint you with the organizational structure that is common in many acute care facilities. Understanding a hospital's organization gives you insight about the proper chain of command, and allows you to address the appropriate personnel with questions, complaints, or suggestions.

The second purpose is to introduce you to the types of acute care facilities that exist, as well as the various departments that may be found within them. As a healthcare worker, familiarity with each department will enhance your confidence and increase your understanding of the function of the hospital.

The third purpose is to emphasize the importance of promoting wellness throughout the hospital environment. Every event, policy, procedure, patient contact, and educational opportunity should lend itself to promoting the patient's complete recovery from his or her present health condition.

Reading Assignment

Read pages 2-1 through 2-20.

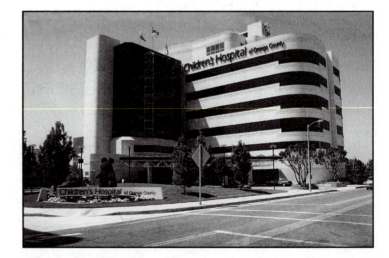

There are many types of acute care hospitals.

Name _____

Date _____

Student Enrichment Activities

Complete the following statements.

1. The organizational structure of a healthcare facility is indicated in the

    _____ _____ _____.

2. A general hospital is a type of _____ _____ hospital.

3. _____ is the branch of medicine that cares for infants, children, and adolescents to 18 years of age.

4. The _____ _____ is the department of the hospital that cares for patients with life or limb-threatening conditions.

5. The first contact the public may have with hospital personnel is usually with the

    _____ _____.

6. _____ is the release of rays in different directions from a common point.

7. The rehabilitation department that is concerned with the restoration of function and the prevention of disability is the _____ _____ Department.

8. In addition to geriatrics, one of the fastest growing areas in healthcare is

    _____ _____.

9. The department of the hospital that treats bone diseases and fractures is

    _____.

10. Reducing the risk of communicable diseases to both the staff and the patients is the responsibility of the _____ _____ _____.

Unscramble the following terms.

11. NICAH FO MAMCOND   _____ _____ _____

12. LRATCICI RECA   _____ - _____

13. CRAYOLADMI   _____

14. CRAFTINION   _____

15. GROOMNI NI   _____ - _____

16. RTNSILITAZIOE   _____

17. SLEWSLEN   _____

Name _____

Date _____

Additional Enrichment Activities

Circle the correct answer.

18. An EKG is a special test that indicates the electrical activity of:

    A. the heart.

    B. the brain.

    C. the muscles.

    D. the kidneys.

19. Therapeutic Services DOES NOT include which department?

    A. Diagnostic Services

    B. Respiratory Therapy

    C. Bio-Engineering

    D. the Pharmacy

20. One of the fastest growing areas of medicine and nursing is:

    A. Neonatal and Pediatrics.

    B. Geriatrics.

    C. Home Health.

    D. Medical Imaging.

21. Nursing Services includes which of the following departments?

    A. Social Services and Discharge Planning

    B. Oncology

    C. Post Anesthesia Care Unit

    D. all of the above

22. Support Services may include all of the following EXCEPT:
    A. Engineering and Maintenance.
    B. Discharge Planning.
    C. the Transportation Department.
    D. Central Supply.

23. An example of an acute care hospital is:
    A. a general hospital
    B. a children's hospital
    C. a rehabilitation hospital
    D. both A and B

24. The hospital department that treats bone diseases and fractures is:
    A. Oncology.
    B. Radiation Therapy.
    C. Orthopedics.
    D. Medical Imaging.

25. Infants, children, and adolescents to 18 years of age usually receive care in the
    _____ Department.
    A. Neonatal
    B. Pediatric
    C. Emergency
    D. none of the above

Name _____

Date _____

Complete the following exercises.

26. Briefly describe the role of the organizational chart and its impact on the overall efficiency of the hospital, as well as its impact on delivery of patient care.

   _____

   _____

   _____

   _____

   _____

   _____

27. List the various departments included under Therapeutic Services and briefly describe each.

   _____

   _____

   _____

   _____

   _____

   _____

   _____

   _____

   _____

   _____

   _____

28. List and briefly describe each of the various departments included under Nursing Services.

_____

_____

_____

_____

_____

_____

_____

_____

_____

_____

_____

_____

_____

_____

_____

_____

_____

29. Describe at least three steps a healthcare worker can take to help promote patient wellness in the hospital.

_____

_____

_____

30. List at least three examples of acute care hospitals.

_____

_____

_____

Name _____

Date _____

The Acute Care Hospital—Puzzle 1

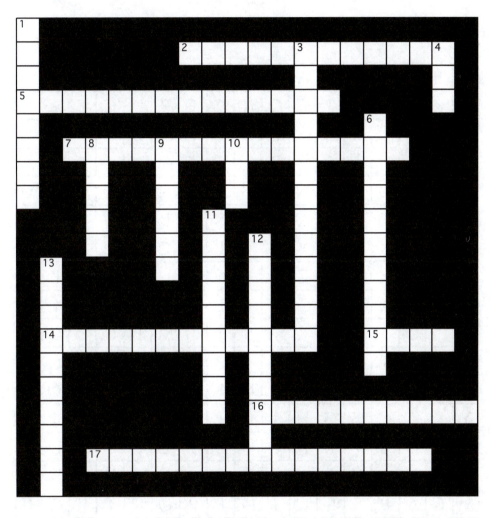

Across

2. The rendering of care to patients with life-threatening conditions (2 words)
5. The organizational structure of a healthcare facility (3 words)
7. Surgery not done in an emergency (2 words)
14. The use of drugs or chemicals to treat or control diseases
15. A plaster or fiberglass mold of a body part
16. See 13 Down
17. Nursing unit that cares for patients recovering from surgery (2 words)

Down

1. A crack or break in a bone
3. The department of the hospital responsible for sterilizing surgical instruments (2 words)
4. The abbreviation for electroencephalogram
6. Deals with the treatment of disorders relating to the skeleton, its joints, and muscles
8. Delivering the fetus from the uterus through the birth canal and out of the mother's body
9. A _____ center is a medical facility that is capable of providing care to critically injured patients 24 hours a day
10. A diagnostic test that measures the electrical activity of the heart
11. The _____ department is an area of an acute care facility that is staffed and equipped to handle patients with life-threatening illnesses or injuries
12. Deals with the problems of aging
13. A heart attack; a condition caused by the blockage of one or more coronary arteries; with 16 Across

Name _____

Date _____

The Acute Care Hospital—Puzzle 2

Find the listed words in the puzzle and circle them. (Contains backwards words.)

E	E	C	I	N	F	A	R	C	T	I	O	N	M	R	E	L
C	K	R	H	I	J	P	Q	A	C	E	P	H	G	E	A	T
H	I	G	U	A	B	W	Z	Z	Q	E	M	B	G	B	M	R
E	A	L	H	T	I	V	B	I	A	E	M	P	O	E	O	A
M	R	K	D	B	C	N	Q	D	C	P	N	R	D	J	R	U
O	S	C	G	Z	A	A	O	N	N	Z	B	I	L	R	J	M
T	C	T	X	M	U	Y	R	F	L	W	C	G	Y	S	V	A
H	I	Y	X	N	P	R	I	F	C	A	U	Y	N	W	K	C
E	R	G	W	Y	Q	Z	T	E	L	O	K	S	K	T	L	E
R	T	Q	F	G	K	X	M	S	J	Q	M	B	Q	B	Q	N
A	A	H	I	O	W	E	U	E	P	Z	F	M	W	Q	N	T
P	I	F	G	R	R	A	N	E	T	K	M	A	X	Q	E
Y	R	T	G	G	U	J	R	T	Q	E	W	T	N	J	R
C	E	D	E	I	X	P	O	I	W	Y	Z	C	U	S	D	I
I	G	N	C	Y	L	A	I	D	R	A	C	O	Y	M	A	E
M	C	A	B	X	S	C	I	D	E	P	O	H	T	R	O	C
Y	L	C	E	N	T	R	A	L	S	U	P	P	L	Y	Y	C

CAST
CENTRAL SUPPLY
CHAIN OF COMMAND
CHEMOTHERAPY
EEG
EKG
EMERGENCY
FRACTURE

GERIATRICS
INFARCTION
LABOR
MEDICAL SURGICAL
MYOCARDIAL
ORTHOPEDICS
TRAUMA CENTER

Chapter Three
Hospital Employees and Medical Staff

Objectives

After completing this chapter you should be able to do the following:

1. Define and correctly spell each of the key terms.

2. Define the term *doctor* and list at least three types of doctors.

3. Identify and discuss at least three clinical allied healthcare positions.

4. Define the phrase *irreversible brain death.*

Key Terms

- high risk
- infertility
- irreversible brain death
- neonate

- organ transplant
- pulmonary medicine
- rheumatology

Chapter Overview

Chapter Three of the textbook discusses the various specialties within the medical profession. There are numerous specialties already, and as technology, skills, and knowledge become more complex, more branches of medicine will evolve.

Time, study, and a sincere desire to learn will be required in order to memorize the many areas of medicine, nursing, and allied health. You will be a positive asset to the hospital and the patients as your skills and knowledge increase! Skillful and knowledgeable employees are one of the key elements in the efficient operation of the healthcare facility.

Reading Assignment

Read pages 3-1 through 3-15.

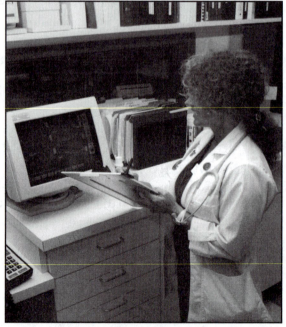

Registered nurses have many different responsibilities, and are subject to all the rules and regulations adopted by the Board of Registered Nursing concerning their scope of practice and licensing requirements.

Name _____

Date _____

Student Enrichment Activities

Complete the following statements.

1. The two types of nurses with whom you will be in contact are _____
   _____ and _____ _____ _____.

2. MD is the accepted abbreviation for _____ _____.

3. A closely related branch of medicine to Family Practice is _____
   _____.

4. Emergency nurses are also called _____ _____ _____.

5. Asthma is a disease that is classified under the branch of _____
   _____.

6. Endoscopy nurses specialize in the field of _____.

7. The branch of medicine concerned with the study of disorders and diseases of the
   joints of the body is called _____.

8. OB-GYN is an accepted abbreviation for _____ and
   _____.

9. Infants younger than the age of 4 weeks are cared for by a specialist in
   _____.

10. The term *plastic* actually means _____ of being _____.

11. Counseling centers specialize in providing assistance to patients with

    _____ _____ .

12. An area of medicine that often raises many ethical questions deals with

    _____ _____ .

Unscramble the following terms.

13. RONCAROY   _____

14. IHHG SIRK   _____   _____

15. TINYFLIRTIE   _____

16. BNRIA EADHT   _____   _____

17. TENAEON   _____

18. STARTNPLAN   _____

19. RONPLAYUM   _____

20. OHGLUEMATORY   _____

Name _____

Date _____

Additional Enrichment Activities

Circle the correct answer.

21. Neurology is a branch of medicine concerned with the study of:

    A. high-risk neonates.

    B. eye diseases, diagnosis, and treatment.

    C. nervous system diseases, and their diagnosis and treatment.

    D. both A and C.

22. The Infection Control Department's main responsibility includes:

    A. reducing the risk of communicable diseases to patients and healthcare workers.

    B. developing and implementing policies and procedures for the CDC.

    C. reporting noncompliance with handwashing procedures to the health department.

    D. monitoring substance abuse in healthcare workers.

23. Members of the healthcare team include:

    A. physicians and nurses.

    B. emergency medical personnel.

    C. allied healthcare workers, including health unit coordinators.

    D. all of the above.

24. The approximate amount of time in school required of a licensed vocational or practical nurse is:

    A. $1^1/_2$ years.

    B. 2-4 years.

    C. 12 months.

    D. 1,020 hours, including clinical work and internships.

25. Internal medicine is a branch of medicine that treats diseases and disorders:

    A. of the female reproductive system.

    B. of oncology.

    C. of the heart and blood vessels.

    D. of adults without surgical intervention.

26. Infertility is an area of medicine practiced by:

    A. a psychiatrist.

    B. an obstetrician and gynecologist.

    C. a gastroenterologist.

    D. an organ transplant specialist.

27. Ophthalmology is:

    A. the study of bone diseases, disorders, and their treatment.

    B. the study of eye, ear, nose, and throat conditions, disorders, and their treatment.

    C. the study of eye diseases, disorders, and their treatment.

    D. both B and C.

28. Gastroenterology is defined as the branch of medicine concerned with the diagnosis and treatment of diseases and disorders of which of the following?

    A. The digestive system.

    B. The hormone secreting ductless glands.

    C. The female reproductive system.

    D. The skin.

29. Otolaryngology is:

    A. the medical specialty concerned with the eyes.

    B. the medical specialty concerned with the nose and throat.

    C. the medical specialty concerned with the ears.

    D. both B and C.

Name _____

Date _____

30. Specialty areas of nursing include:
    A. obstetrics and gynecology.
    B. cardiology.
    C. critical care.
    D. all of the above.

Complete the following exercises.

31. Briefly describe the following.
    A. primary care nursing:_____

    _____

    B. team nursing care: _____

    _____

32. Describe the roles of the following allied healthcare professionals and list the title of
    the position of the person who is legally responsible for providing direct supervision.
    A. CNA: _____

    _____

    _____

    _____

    B. MA: _____

    _____

    _____

    _____

33. Briefly describe the following medical specialties and the type of nurse specialist that is associated with each of them.

A. rheumatology: _____

_____

B. neonatology: _____

_____

C. gastroenterology: _____

_____

D. cardiology: _____

_____

E. gerontology: _____

_____

F. urology: _____

_____

Name _____

Date _____

Hospital Employees and Medical Staff—Puzzle 1

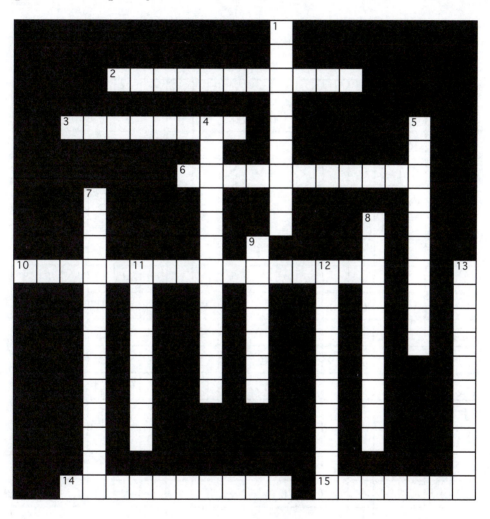

Across

2. The diminished ability or inability to produce children
3. Pertaining to the heart and its blood vessels
6. Concerned with caring for infants from birth to 1 month
10. Area of medicine that studies diseases of the esophagus, stomach, and intestinal tract
14. Branch of medicine that focuses on specific problems concerning the uterus, fallopian tubes, ovaries, cervix, vagina, and breasts
15. Manual and operative procedures used to repair injuries, correct deformities and defects, and diagnose certain diseases

Down

1. Of or relating to the lungs
4. Concerned with disorders and diseases of the joints of the body
5. Study of the mind and behavior patterns
7. Deals with disorders and diseases of the eye
8. Most premedical students take courses in advanced sciences such as chemistry, physics, biology, anatomy, and _____
9. Deals with dysfunctions of the urinary tract and the male reproductive system
11. Concerned with the diagnosis and treatment of tumors
12. Provides care to pregnant patients both before and up to 6 weeks after the delivery of the baby
13. Deals with the diagnosing, treatment, and prevention of conditions of the heart and its blood vessels

Name _____

Date _____

Hospital Employees and Medical Staff—Puzzle 2

Find the listed words in the puzzle and circle them. (Contains backwards words.)

C	D	V	J	L	I	Y	Y	G	O	L	O	R	H	P	E	N	Y
P	O	Y	P	I	B	L	E	Z	L	J	J	X	V	L	F	R	C
S	H	R	G	N	X	B	O	S	K	F	K	V	V	U	A	A	V
Y	V	T	O	O	C	D	T	V	N	Y	U	G	B	N	R	P	O
C	O	W	A	N	L	A	Y	E	Z	O	C	C	O	D	X	Z	Q
H	W	Q	H	E	A	O	T	S	P	X	M	M	I	L	Y	D	D
O	V	O	A	K	D	R	R	F	O	H	L	A	Y	J	A	H	C
L	P	Z	B	L	T	N	Y	U	Y	U	C	U	Y	N	N	T	T
O	U	V	L	Q	T	J	I	J	P	Y	J	O	G	B	Z	L	K
G	T	I	V	E	P	I	G	A	G	N	C	M	N	U	T	N	L
Y	N	P	V	Z	Q	W	H	O	R	O	L	N	C	W	Y	N	N
Q	N	Q	V	D	B	I	L	T	Z	B	N	G	W	M	Y	G	W
P	N	E	Y	S	G	O	U	U	I	M	Z	C	D	F	H	M	P
M	O	R	I	H	C	A	W	P	B	X	A	D	O	G	C	Z	K
O	I	C	R	E	T	S	K	A	C	N	H	N	N	L	R	J	I
Q	N	I	N	R	Z	V	K	Y	E	C	E	L	A	D	O	L	A
I	S	Y	C	Y	V	F	E	L	M	O	W	W	A	S	Q	G	W
K	G	H	M	V	C	A	B	H	B	X	O	G	G	R	F	T	Y

BRAIN DEATH   NEPHROLOGY
CARDIAC   ONCOLOGY
CORONARY   PSYCHOLOGY
GYNECOLOGY   PULMONARY
HIGH RISK   UROLOGY

Chapter Four
The Allied Health Worker, the Law, and Professional Ethics

Objectives

After completing this chapter you should be able to
do the following:

1. Define and correctly spell each of the key terms.

2. Name and describe both allied health professional organizations.

3. Explain the term *ethics*.

4. Describe the Patient's Bill of Rights.

5. Name and explain each of the four parts of the patient/healthcare provider contract.

6. Identify and describe at least four kinds of intentional torts.

7. Identify at least seven ways to decrease your chances of being sued.

8. Identify at least four guidelines to follow when witnessing a consent.

9. Describe the legal aspects of AIDS and confidentiality.

10. Define and state the purpose of advance directives.

Key Terms

- abandonment
- advance directives
- battery
- breach of duty to act
- contract
- damages
- duty to act
- ethics
- healthcare provider

- Health Occupations Students of America (HOSA)
- malpractice
- negligence
- patient advocate
- Patient's Bill of Rights
- privileged information
- proximate cause
- scope of practice
- tort

Chapter Overview

Unfortunately, society in general does not hesitate to initiate a lawsuit against a healthcare provider. Providing hands-on care, documenting care given to patients, obtaining legal consent, caring for patients with a diagnosis of AIDS or HIV positive, and maintaining confidentiality are some of the areas in which lawsuits occur. The most frequent complaints concern the lack of time the healthcare provider spent with the patient and the lack of information provided to the patient by the healthcare provider. Chapter Four of the textbook is dedicated to providing information regarding a healthcare worker's legal scope of practice, ethics, and responsibilities. All healthcare workers MUST be knowledgeable regarding their legal responsibilities, restrictions, and rights as well as those of the patient.

As the patient advocate, you have the responsibility to keep yourself educated and well-skilled. Although there are several areas in which lawsuits can occur, treating patients with kindness, consideration, and respect may greatly decrease your chances of being named as a defendant!

Reading Assignment

Read pages 4-1 through 4-14.

Laws define the categories of work that healthcare workers legally may and may not do; but ethics, which set principles even higher than the law, are just as important.

Name _____

Date _____

Student Enrichment Activities

Complete the following statements.

1. Healthcare workers act as the _____ _____.

2. Healthcare professionals must never exceed their legal _____ _____
_____.

3. Principles and moral decisions are determined by one's _____.

4. The document that identifies the basic rights of all patients is the _____
_____ _____ _____.

5. The professional relationship between the healthcare provider and the patient is a
_____.

6. The four items that constitute a breach of contract are:
_____, _____,
_____, and _____.

7. The two types of lawsuits common to the healthcare field are _____
and _____.

8. A private or civil wrong against another person is a _____.

9. Healthcare workers know special information about patients. This information is
_____.

10. _____ confidentiality and testing remains controversial.

Unscramble the following terms.

11. STICHE   _____

12. TRAMICPLACE   _____

13. CROCTNAT   _____

14. APTNIET AVDCOTAE   _____ _____

15. ROTT   _____

16. TRAYBET   _____

17. ILENGCENGE   _____

18. SLATUSA   _____

19. ILCIV LWA   _____ _____

20. STIEPOINDO   _____

Name _____

Date _____

Additional Enrichment Activities

Circle the correct answer.

21. Which of the following are excerpts from the Patient's Bill of Rights?
    A. The patient is entitled to know the names of the healthcare providers treating him.
    B. The patient has a right to refuse participation in research projects.
    C. Case discussion, consultation, examination, and treatment should be conducted discreetly.
    D. all of the above

22. Negligence by a professional is:
    A. battery.
    B. defamation of character.
    C. malpractice.
    D. fraud and misrepresentation.

23. Privileged information is:
    A. information available only to physicians.
    B. information available only to the media.
    C. patient information that can be freely discussed.
    D. special, confidential information about patients.

24. A written law that defines certain categories of work that healthcare workers legally may and may not do is called a:
    A. job description.
    B. scope of practice.
    C. patient advocate.
    D. subpoena.

25. A type of intentional tort is:

    A. proximate cause.

    B. damages.

    C. invasion of privacy.

    D. none of the above.

26. A written, signed consent must be obtained from a patient who is going to be tested for:

    A. HIV.

    B. hepatitis B.

    C. sexually transmitted diseases.

    D. syphilis.

27. Protocols are:

    A. statutes of limitations.

    B. testimonies.

    C. scopes of practice.

    D. established rules for a particular procedure.

28. A contractual relationship includes:

    A. duty to act and compensation.

    B. relevance.

    C. mutual agreement.

    D. all of the above.

29. All are parts of a contract except:

    A. duty to act and relevance.

    B. compensation.

    C. damages and proximate cause.

    D. mutual agreement.

Name _____

Date _____

30. Intentional withholding of information from a patient by a healthcare worker to cover up a mistake is called:

   A. fraud and misrepresentation.

   B. malpractice.

   C. defamation of character.

   D. none of the above.

Complete the following exercises.

31. Define the following terms.

   A. incompetent: _____

   _____

   B. plaintiff: _____

   _____

   C. defendant: _____

   _____

   D. respondeat superior: _____

   _____

   E. statute: _____

   _____

   F. deposition: _____

   _____

32. Explain the phrase *scope of practice*.

   _____

   _____

   _____

   _____

   _____

33. Discuss ethics and how they relate to rules, regulations, and laws.

_____

_____

_____

_____

34. List at least six patient rights as contained within the *Patient's Bill of Rights.*

_____

_____

_____

_____

_____

_____

_____

_____

_____

_____

35. Provide an explanation of the four elements of a contract.

_____

_____

_____

_____

36. Provide an explanation of the four items that must be proven in a lawsuit.

_____

_____

_____

_____

Name _____

Date _____

The Allied Health Worker, the Law, and Professional Ethics—Puzzle 1

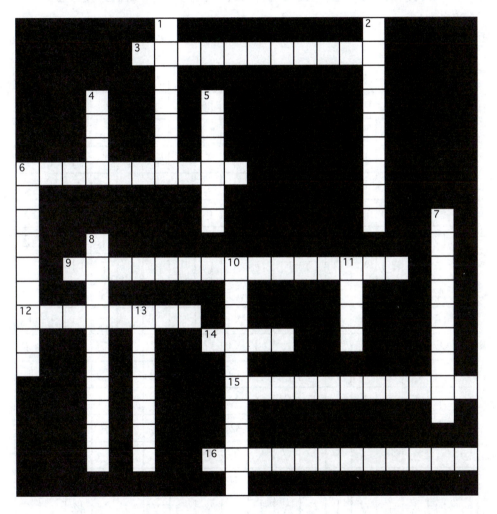

Across

3. Professional misconduct or lack of professional skill that results in injury to the patient
6. Discussion of a person that damages that person's reputation
9. Latin for "it speaks for itself" (3 words)
12. See 1 down
14. Vocational Industrial Clubs of America
15. The termination of supervision of a patient by a physician without adequate written notice or the patient's consent
16. Statements by professional organizations regarding standards to be used to govern decisions made by professional healthcare providers (3 words)

Down

1. An individual who supports and pleads the cause of the patient; with 12 Across
2. A statement, given under oath in a courtroom, providing details of a particular incident
4. Health Occupations Students of America
5. A major crime that is punishable by a greater means than a misdemeanor
6. The legal responsibility to provide care within the scope of practice (3 words)
7. A final decision from a court
8. Testimony given under oath concerning the events of a particular incident
10. A lawsuit
11. A private or civil wrong against another person or their property
13. The threat of an immediate harmful or offensive contact, without actual commission of the act

Name _____

Date _____

The Allied Health Worker, the Law, and Professional Ethics—Puzzle 2

Find the listed words in the puzzle and circle them. (Contains backwards words.)

O	C	K	L	K	D	R	P	N	O	I	T	A	G	I	T	I	L
I	F	Y	K	W	J	X	D	F	F	D	T	T	C	U	T	M	K
P	K	G	M	H	B	F	Z	T	X	M	N	J	D	T	H	K	W
G	G	A	X	B	B	J	G	P	T	E	L	Y	Y	J	H	Y	R
B	X	D	B	K	E	K	I	N	M	L	S	P	I	F	A	J	C
Q	O	M	Q	Y	H	P	E	N	O	C	U	T	O	O	E	O	X
K	D	R	O	O	T	H	O	T	D	I	O	A	A	J	X	A	Z
C	Y	C	O	X	P	D	N	P	T	U	T	N	S	T	U	B	R
W	W	T	L	A	N	A	L	C	U	E	T	I	T	S	U	H	Y
D	G	S	A	A	D	A	I	T	M	J	S	Y	S	R	A	T	H
J	W	L	B	N	I	V	A	H	M	V	S	T	T	O	A	H	E
P	N	A	E	N	I	N	S	L	D	L	D	M	I	O	P	C	M
Z	J	F	T	L	E	E	S	M	X	T	V	F	Z	M	A	E	T
W	E	I	L	O	G	C	K	L	V	I	Z	W	E	B	O	C	D
D	F	A	P	A	I	A	V	X	T	L	A	M	M	Q	N	N	T
F	W	B	M	H	A	X	E	S	E	W	P	S	C	E	G	S	Y
N	U	A	T	V	I	C	A	T	L	Y	Q	Y	U	L	K	I	C
S	D	E	A	D	A	P	Z	V	E	Q	J	Z	Y	T	R	O	T

ABANDONMENT	ETHICS
ASSAULT	LITIGATION
CIVIL LAW	PLAINTIFF
CONTRACT	STATUTE
DAMAGES	SUBPOENA
DEFENDANT	TESTIMONY
DEPOSITION	TORT
DUTY TO ACT	VICA

Chapter Five
Understanding the Patient as a Person

Objectives

After completing this chapter you should be able to
do the following:

1. Define and correctly spell each of the key terms.

2. List the seven life stages.

3. Identify the four aspects of growth and development affected in each life stage.

4. List at least four characteristics of each life stage.

5. Identify at least three causes of stress that may affect an individual.

6. Describe the steps that may lead to a crisis situation.

7. List and describe the five stages in the dying process.

8. Explain hospice care.

9. Define the phrase *right to die.*

Key Terms

- Alzheimer's disease
- coping mechanisms
- culture
- custom
- death

- Elisabeth Kubler-Ross
- hospice
- life stage
- palliative
- right to die

Chapter Overview

When providing patient care, it is easy to become so involved with the tasks you perform, that kindness, empathy, and compassion toward the patient may be lost. Therefore, the main theme of this chapter is THE PATIENT IS A PERSON. Understanding the seven life stages that all people experience enhances the ability of the healthcare worker to more clearly understand the actions and reactions of the patient and/or the family.

Death is a natural part of life. As healthcare workers understand the needs and desires of the dying patient and his or her family, supportive care becomes a natural response. The five stages of the dying process, along with the seven life stages, paint a complex picture of people. Always remember that patients are people, and basic needs and life's responsibilities do not end with hospitalization!

Practice courtesy, kindness, compassion, and sincerity toward one another in and out of the classroom. This will naturally carry over to your home and to your patients.

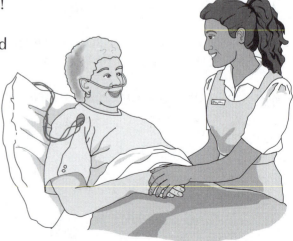

Reading Assignment

Read pages 5-1 through 5-18.

Compassion is vital when dealing with patients and their loved ones.

Name _____

Date _____

Student Enrichment Activities

Complete the following statements.

1. It is not unusual for the elderly to spend approximately _____ of their income on healthcare.

2. There are _____ different life stages throughout one's life span.

3. In a healthy life span, total dependency on others for all physical, mental, emotional, and social needs usually occurs during _____.

4. It is estimated that within the next 10 years, 1 out of 2 people over the age of 80 will be affected by some stage of _____ _____.

5. During the _____ _____ stage, the social skills are influenced by both the parents and the peers.

6. Substance abuse and suicide can be enormous problems during _____.

7. Establishing a career, selecting a marital partner, and determining a particular lifestyle often occur during _____ _____.

8. Inadequate coping mechanisms result in a negative occurrence of _____.

9. Two hospital departments that may be valuable resources during times of stress are _____ _____ and _____ _____.

10. _____ _____ _____ is a well-known authority on death and dying.

11. An important supportive service offering care and counseling to dying patients and their families is _____ _____.

12. A controversial issue concerning the rights of patients is the _____ _____ _____.

Unscramble the following terms.

13. FILE TESAGS   _____ _____

14. GIRTH OT IDE   _____ _____ _____

15. LIVEATALIP   _____

16. SHOPICE   _____

17. LIZAREMESH SEASIDE   _____ _____

18. TRUELUC   _____

19. UBPRETY   _____

20. GINPCO SCHEMAMIN   _____ _____

Name _____

Date _____

Additional Enrichment Activities

Circle the correct answer.

21. Dr. Elisabeth Kubler-Ross is best known for her work with:

    A. Alzheimer's Disease.

    B. life stages.

    C. death and dying.

    D. none of the above.

22. Almost 50% of the personal income of people over the age of 85 is spent on:

    A. transportation.

    B. healthcare.

    C. food.

    D. medications.

23. The life stage known as early adulthood includes those between the ages of:

    A. 20 and 40 years old.

    B. 18 and 35 years old.

    C. 25 and 45 years old.

    D. none of the above.

24. Two hospital departments that may assist the patient with stressful concerns are:

    A. Social Services and Discharge Planning.

    B. Rehabilitation and Physical Therapy.

    C. Speech and Occupational Therapy.

    D. the Pharmacy and Dietary Department.

25. Striking out at anyone who happens to be available and showing hostility and bitterness is most characteristic of this stage of the dying process:

    A. denial.

    B. bargaining.

    C. anger.

    D. depression.

26. Two dangerous eating disorders experienced during adolescence are:

    A. regression and depression.

    B. hyperactivity and bipolar disease.

    C. bulimia and anorexia nervosa.

    D. manic-depressive disorder and schizophrenia.

Complete the following exercises.

27. Describe the following life stages.

    A. early childhood: _____

    _____

    _____

    B. middle adulthood: _____

    _____

    _____

    C. late adulthood: _____

    _____

    _____

    D. infancy: _____

    _____

    _____

Name _____

Date _____

28. Identify and describe each of the five stages of the dying process.

_____

_____

_____

_____

_____

_____

_____

_____

_____

29. Define the term *coping mechanism,* and list several methods of coping a patient may utilize during hospitalization.

_____

_____

_____

_____

_____

30. Define and describe the following life stages.

A. adolescence: _____

_____

_____

_____

B. early adulthood: _____

_____

_____

_____

31. Identify the four aspects of growth and development that are affected by each life stage.

_____

_____

_____

32. Briefly describe the projected impact of healthcare issues from infancy to geriatrics.

_____

_____

_____

_____

_____

_____

Name _____

Date _____

Understanding the Patient as a Person—Puzzle 1

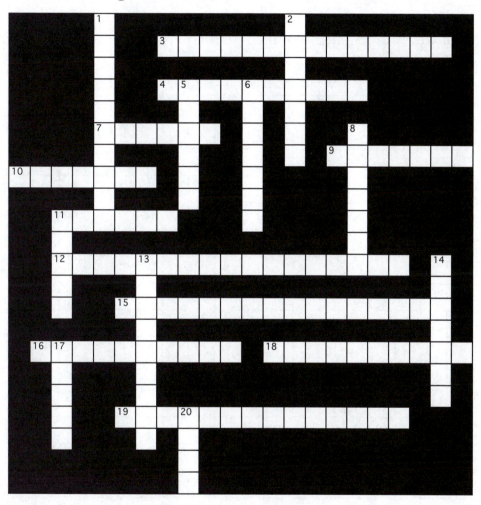

Across

3. Excessive use of chemicals, drugs, or alcohol (2 words)
4. Final stage of the dying process
7. When events or circumstances challenge or exceed one's coping mechanisms
9. The skills and arts of a given people at a given time
10. The voluntary ending of one's life
11. The first stage of the dying process
12. Causes irreversible memory loss and physical deterioration, commonly seen in late adulthood (2 words)
15. The methods by which an individual adjusts or adapts to a challenge or stressful situation (2 words)
16. The third stage of the dying process
18. Concerns the right of a terminally ill patient to request that no life-sustaining measures be taken (3 words)
19. Describes children between the ages of 1 and 6 years old (2 words)

Down

1. The fourth stage of the dying process
2. Describes babies from birth to 1 year of age
5. A tradition or usual practice of a particular people or social group
6. When males and females become capable of reproduction
8. A mental illness characterized by overeating binges typically followed by voluntary vomiting, fasting, or induced diarrhea
11. The end of life as indicated by the permanent cessation of all vital functions
13. Referring to one's feelings
14. An agency offering care and counseling to dying patients and their families
17. The second stage of the dying process
20. The quality or state of being alive

Name _____

Date _____

Understanding the Patient as a Person—Puzzle 2

Find the listed words in the puzzle and circle them. (Contains backwards words.)

O	N	M	T	P	V	X	Z	U	J	W	O	T	V	P	X	T	L
S	K	F	I	X	P	X	G	E	F	Q	Y	G	U	L	N	S	I
A	T	W	G	N	L	S	G	O	O	T	W	B	E	E	Z	U	G
U	S	R	F	T	W	X	X	S	W	B	E	C	M	L	Y	X	K
N	R	O	E	Y	H	G	Z	D	A	R	I	P	R	H	S	P	Y
Q	U	U	V	S	A	B	X	O	T	P	O	S	N	H	X	C	T
X	X	Q	E	R	S	W	J	Y	S	L	P	N	Q	O	S	Q	U
P	V	X	A	C	E	Z	Z	O	E	W	U	V	F	E	F	S	I
V	F	W	X	X	N	N	H	V	P	W	B	V	I	K	Z	E	N
X	X	O	A	A	D	E	E	S	T	Q	M	G	L	Z	Y	G	O
L	O	H	M	M	D	D	C	A	E	S	Z	A	L	I	P	A	I
A	U	A	J	H	L	O	Q	S	I	E	G	G	Q	S	K	T	S
C	W	A	C	A	O	E	X	C	E	X	D	P	L	K	U	S	S
A	X	W	I	G	G	J	O	H	H	L	E	I	B	U	R	E	E
M	O	C	J	F	M	Y	N	A	C	E	O	R	C	E	G	F	R
F	O	Q	T	V	L	F	K	B	J	P	H	D	O	I	F	I	P
S	S	O	X	L	D	A	X	S	P	X	L	Y	A	N	U	L	E
M	V	P	D	E	J	L	A	N	O	I	T	O	M	E	A	S	D

ADOLESCENCE

ANOREXIA

DEPRESSION

DEVELOPMENT

EMOTIONAL

HOSPICE

LIFE STAGES

NERVOSA

PUBERTY

SOCIAL

STRESS

SUICIDE

Chapter Six
Communication Skills

Objectives

After completing this chapter you should be able to
do the following:

1.   Define and correctly spell each of the key terms.

2.   Identify examples of verbal and nonverbal
     communication skills.

3.   Name at least three factors that influence the transmission
     of a message.

4.   Name at least three factors that influence the receipt of
     a message.

5.   Describe each of the five levels of Maslow's Hierarchy of
     Needs and the factors that may affect each level.

6.   Describe at least three defense mechanisms and give
     examples of each.

7.   List five rules of proper telephone etiquette.

Key Terms

- Abraham Maslow
- communication
- defense mechanisms
- Maslow's Hierarchy of Needs
- need

- nonverbal
- receiver
- sender
- significant other
- verbal

Chapter Overview

The main purpose of Chapter Six is to help you refine your verbal and nonverbal communication skills. In modern society, basic spoken communication often is substituted by other forms of communication such as faxes, on-line postings, alpha pagers, various codes, and computer screens. Nonverbal skills, like body language, also play an important role in communication.

Since unspoken communication often replaces the spoken word, learning to effectively communicate with patients, family and friends, and professional colleagues is of the utmost importance for nurturing relationships. Remember—thoughtful, truthful, and excellent communication (both verbal and nonverbal) is often the key to avoiding a lawsuit!

Reading Assignment

Read pages 6-1 through 6-18.

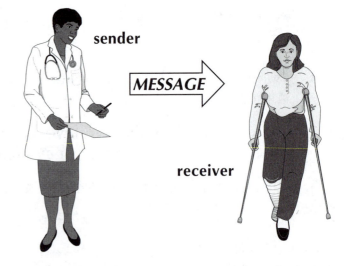

Communication involves a message and at least two people: a sender and a receiver.

Name _____

Date _____

Student Enrichment Activities

Complete the following statements.

1. The three parts of any communication are the _____, the _____, and the _____.

2. Body language and tactile stimulation are examples of _____ _____.

3. The effective sending of a message is enhanced when _____ and _____ are kept to a minimum.

4. Accurate information is best obtained by asking _____ questions.

5. _____ listening requires a conscious effort from the receiver.

6. Five categories of human needs were identified by _____ _____.

7. Two methods of satisfying human needs are _____ and _____.

8. A category of indirect methods of meeting human needs is called _____ _____.

9. When placing callers on hold, remember that _____ is the key.

10. Two examples of communication, other than the telephone, are
    _____ and _____.

11. Computers are the communication _____ of the
    healthcare facility.

Unscramble the following terms.

12. MARHABA SMOWAL   _____ _____

13. UNTIMAICOMCON   _____

14. SNEEFED SCHEMASMIN   _____ _____

15. CHRYARIEH   _____

16. CRIEVERE   _____

17. DRESEN   _____

18. BLAVER   _____

19. XYLASUITE   _____

Name _____

Date _____

Additional Enrichment Activities

Circle the correct answer.

20. The psychologist given credit for identifying essential human needs was:
    A. Elisabeth Kubler-Ross.
    B. Paul L. Marlowe.
    C. Abraham Maslow.
    D. Rudenz Douthat.

21. Projection is a type of:
    A. compensation mechanism.
    B. defense mechanism.
    C. adaptation mechanism.
    D. none of the above.

22. Self-actualization is:
    A. a form of daydreaming.
    B. the highest level of human need.
    C. achieved during young adulthood.
    D. a life stage.

23. Active listening is:
    A. making a conscious effort to hear and understand what the sender is saying.
    B. listening to conversation while working.
    C. rephrasing the received message.
    D. clarifying the sender's message.

24. Before the message is accepted and believed, the receiver must:

    A. practice clarification.

    B. use the active listening skill.

    C. rephrase the message.

    D. have confidence and trust in the sender of the message.

25. The verbal or nonverbal exchange of messages, ideas, thoughts, feelings, and information is:

    A. a defense mechanism.

    B. a coping mechanism.

    C. terminology.

    D. communication.

Complete the following exercises.

26. List and explain each of the ten guidelines for proper telephone etiquette.

    _____

    _____

    _____

    _____

    _____

    _____

    _____

    _____

    _____

    _____

    _____

    _____

    _____

Name _____

Date _____

27. Define each of the following.

    A. rationalization: _____

    _____

    B. projection: _____

    _____

    C. compensation: _____

    _____

    D. displacement: _____

    _____

    Collectively these are called _____ _____.

28. Describe several factors that might interfere with the transmission and receipt of the intended message.

    _____

    _____

    _____

    _____

    _____

    _____

    _____

    _____

    _____

    _____

29. Describe the two types of questions generally used by healthcare workers.

    _____

    _____

    _____

30. List and describe each level of Maslow's Hierarchy of Needs.

_____

_____

_____

_____

_____

_____

_____

_____

_____

_____

31. List seven types of communication devices and describe how each is used.

_____

_____

_____

_____

_____

_____

_____

_____

_____

_____

_____

_____

_____

_____

_____

Name _____

Date _____

Communication Skills—Puzzle 1

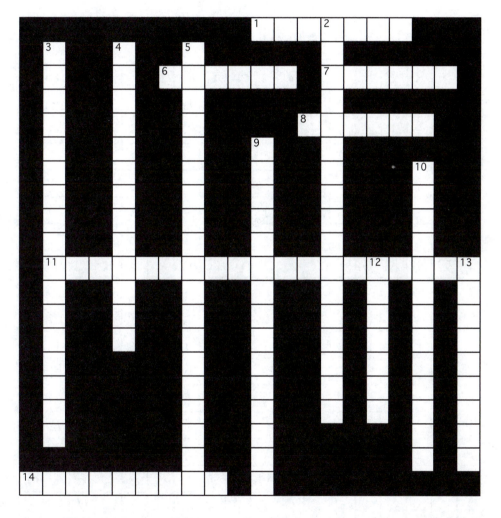

Across

1. A decrease in size or wasting away usually due to lack of use
6. The person who attempts to transmit information to another person or a group of people
7. Refers to one's value, worth, or importance
8. Spoken communication
11. A type of question that restricts the answer to a "yes" or "no" (3 words)
14. One aspect of the need for love and affection

Down

2. A type of question in which the answer is not restricted to a "yes" or "no" answer (3 words)
3. Methods of unconscious behavior that help people in coping and adapting to life (2 words)
4. Psychologist credited with a theory of motivation that identified five levels of human needs (2 words)
5. What the receiver says to indicate to the sender how a message was heard and received (2 words)
9. Making a conscious effort to hear what the sender is communicating (2 words)
10. A communication skill that prompts the sender to explain any part of the message about which the receiver was unclear
12. Stimulation through touch, sight, taste, smell, and hearing
13. A form of communication that involves body language, tactile stimulation, and facial expressions

Name _____

Date _____

Communication Skills—Puzzle 2

Find the listed words in the puzzle and circle them. (Contains backwards words.)

O	N	R	J	P	E	E	V	I	T	C	E	L	F	E	R	E	R
P	P	O	Y	V	R	K	Y	Q	C	M	U	X	K	R	S	E	L
R	M	E	I	H	Y	H	B	A	O	O	P	Y	G	T	V	O	K
O	Q	I	N	T	P	M	W	B	V	J	B	M	E	I	V	P	G
J	L	Y	Q	E	A	O	O	N	D	D	Y	E	E	E	C	Y	L
E	W	J	P	P	N	Z	R	F	F	H	M	C	A	Y	B	Q	S
C	R	F	A	D	F	D	I	T	P	K	E	N	F	I	V	L	M
T	O	M	K	B	E	A	E	L	A	R	D	V	S	R	Z	I	B
I	T	O	M	W	P	Z	T	D	A	A	Y	L	V	X	N	Z	K
O	F	N	T	P	Z	F	Y	S	F	U	W	D	V	P	L	O	S
N	L	F	N	B	S	G	E	F	C	I	T	R	Z	E	P	E	T
J	A	S	V	N	Q	X	E	W	X	J	N	C	O	Y	E	H	O
K	B	L	J	S	U	C	N	J	N	P	D	A	S	J	Q	B	
F	R	W	J	A	T	L	K	G	B	U	O	B	I	F	N	R	V
M	E	Z	L	I	T	I	K	V	U	G	W	C	H	R	L	E	D
P	V	I	O	C	E	R	D	H	J	J	V	G	H	Q	E	E	S
Y	T	N	A	W	E	C	S	Z	Z	A	Q	I	Y	W	V	C	S
Y	C	L	O	S	E	D	E	N	D	E	D	R	E	N	H	I	T

ATROPHY	RECEIVER
CLOSED ENDED	REFLECTIVE
ESTEEM	SELF ACTUALIZATION
INDIRECT	SENSOR
LOVE AND AFFECTION	SEXUALITY
OPEN ENDED	VERBAL
PROJECTION	

Chapter Seven
The Safe Workplace

Objectives

After completing this chapter you should be able to do the following:

1. Define and correctly spell each of the key terms.

2. Identify the three natural curves of the back.

3. Name at least four basic guidelines for proper body mechanics, and explain why using them is important.

4. List at least three rules for the use of siderails.

5. Identify three hazards that may result in falls.

6. Name at least two restrictions for patients who smoke.

7. List at least five ways to reduce the risk of electrical shock.

8. Identify at least three rules to follow for chemical safety.

9. Describe the steps that should be taken if a fire occurs.

10. Explain how to use a fire extinguisher.

Key Terms

- alignment
- body mechanics
- cardiopulmonary resuscitation (CPR)

- hazard communication label
- Material Safety Data Sheet
- range of motion
- sudden death

Chapter Overview

The information contained within Chapter Seven is designed to help you establish and maintain a safe working environment. It is not solely the employer's responsibility to provide a safe workplace; the employees also have responsibility, as well as liability, in this important area.

The patients and their loved ones depend on healthcare workers to care for them in a safe environment and to protect them from safety hazards. This includes maintaining the working order of equipment, using proper body mechanics, and knowing how to perform procedures properly.

Reading Assignment

Read pages 7-1 through 7-22.

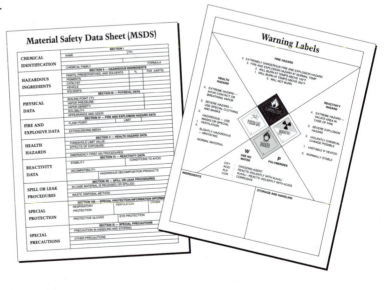

As a responsible employee, you must be aware of possible safety hazards such as dangerous chemicals, and exercise proper judgement while working.

Name _____

Date _____

Student Enrichment Activities

Complete the following statements.

1. The three natural curves of the back are the _____, the _____, and the _____ curves.

2. The thirty-three bones of the spinal column are called _____.

3. The muscles of the _____, _____, _____, and _____ help support the spine. Keeping them strong and flexible can help prevent serious injury to the spine.

4. Self-injury is at its lowest risk when proper _____ _____ are used.

5. Two serious diseases capable of being transmitted to healthcare workers through dirty needles or sharp objects are _____ and _____.

6. During a patient transfer, the _____ is the *load* or *object*.

7. Many lawsuits stem from healthcare workers NOT using _____.

8. One of the keys to the prevention of falls is never leave the patient _____.

9. Patients must never be allowed to smoke when _____ is near.

10. All hospital personnel must complete a course in cardiopulmonary

    _____.

11. The possibility of _____ _____ always exists

    when using equipment.

12. The most common type of chemical injury is a _____.

13. Where there is _____, there is _____.

Unscramble the following terms.

14. TIMEGLANN   _____

15. OBYD SCHEMACIN   _____ _____

16. RICARDOPLAYONUM   _____

17. ISTARTSCIONUE   _____

18. DEDSUN HATED   _____ _____

19. ROCHATIC   _____

20. ICRAVECL   _____

Name _____

Date _____

Additional Enrichment Activities

Circle the correct answer.

21. Electric shock can result from:

    A. the use of malfunctioning equipment.

    B. the use of damaged electrical cords.

    C. the use of inappropriate electrical prongs.

    D. all of the above.

22. When using a fire extinguisher, DO NOT:

    A. direct the spray at the base of the fire.

    B. pull the pin—this should remain intact.

    C. hold the extinguisher at an angle.

    D. hold the extinguisher upright.

23. Each hospital bed and gurney is equipped with:

    A. siderails.

    B. a call light and intercom system.

    C. a storage basket for patient belongings.

    D. an O_2 tank.

24. The most common industrial injuries among healthcare workers are:

    A. needle sticks.

    B. back injuries.

    C. industrial illnesses.

    D. both A and B.

25. A needle stick may be capable of transmitting:

    A. tuberculosis.

    B. AIDS.

    C. hepatitis.

    D. both B and C.

26. The are _____ thoracic vertebrae in the human back.

    A. twelve

    B. seven

    C. five

    D. thirty-three

27. The purpose of a disc in the spine is to:

    A. maintain proper alignment.

    B. act as a shock absorber.

    C. maintain the three natural curves.

    D. prevent injuries.

Complete the following exercises.

28. Briefly describe the anatomy of a healthy back.

    _____

    _____

    _____

    _____

    _____

    _____

    _____

Name _____

Date _____

29. List eight guidelines that may help prevent patient falls and injuries to healthcare workers.

_____

_____

_____

_____

_____

_____

_____

_____

_____

30. List the seven guidelines for avoiding chemical injuries.

_____

_____

_____

_____

_____

_____

_____

_____

31. Define *Material Safety Data Sheets* and describe the information they contain.

_____

_____

_____

_____

_____

32. Describe the proper uses of each of the following.

    A. Class A fire extinguisher: _____

    _____

    B. Class B fire extinguisher: _____

    _____

    C. Class C fire extinguisher: _____

    _____

    D. Class D fire extinguisher: _____

    _____

33. Explain the purpose of CPR.

_____

_____

_____

34. List nine guidelines that may help reduce the risk of electric shock.

_____

_____

_____

_____

_____

_____

_____

_____

_____

35. Describe four safety steps to take when providing care to patients who smoke.

_____

_____

_____

_____

Name _____

Date _____

36. List at least four types of healthcare workers at risk to acquire a needle-stick injury.

_____

_____

37. List six guidelines to help prevent back injuries.

_____

_____

_____

_____

_____

_____

38. Describe the procedural steps for the following.

  A. Transferring a patient from the bed to a gurney:

_____

_____

_____

_____

_____

_____

_____

_____

_____

_____

_____

_____

B. Transferring a patient from the bed to a wheelchair:

_____

_____

_____

_____

_____

_____

_____

_____

_____

_____

_____

_____

_____

Name _____

Date _____

The Safe Workplace—Puzzle 1

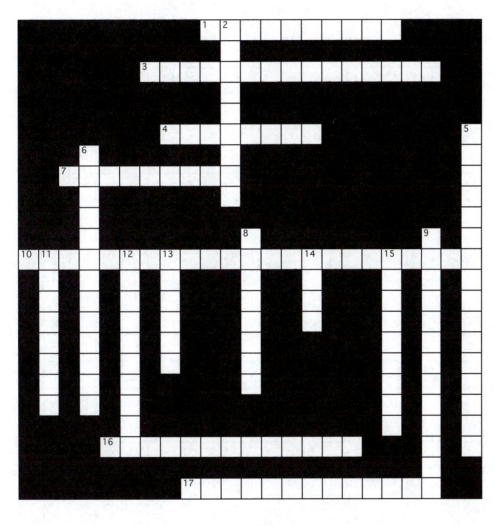

Across

1. A jagged tear in the flesh
3. The basic lifesaving procedure that is done in the event of a cardiac arrest; with 9 Down
4. A substance capable of causing injury either through direct contact on the skin or by the inhalation of gaseous fumes
7. A soft tissue injury caused by seepage of blood into tissue; a bruise
10. An official document that identifies all the chemicals used in a specific department (4 words)
16. An extreme stimulation of the nerves by the passage of current through the body (2 words)
17. The extent to which a joint can move (3 words)

Down

2. The positioning of parts in a straight line
5. A canister filled with chemicals to combat different types of fires (2 words)
6. The efficient and safe use of the body during activity (2 words)
8. Pertaining to the upper portion of the spine
9. Revive or bring back to life; See 3 Across
11. An unforeseen, unfortunate occurrence; See 12 Down
12. An injury sustained while working; with 11 Down
13. The lower back between the thorax and the pelvis
14. A cartilaginous cushion between the vertebrae
15. Devices on a bed or gurney used to prevent a patient from falling

Name _____

Date _____

The Safe Workplace—Puzzle 2

Find the listed words in the puzzle and circle them. (Contains backwards words.)

V	H	U	A	Q	O	X	Z	L	A	C	I	V	R	E	C	C	P
C	H	E	M	I	C	A	L	D	I	T	S	D	F	R	P	V	P
N	K	H	O	T	T	B	F	G	M	Z	O	R	L	R	C	E	P
L	O	R	E	D	X	D	V	W	Q	Z	Y	U	F	O	T	R	F
N	Y	F	M	V	S	R	Q	C	N	A	P	E	N	V	H	T	J
C	O	T	G	V	C	S	O	R	W	M	E	T	H	N	O	E	D
D	O	I	E	C	F	N	Z	X	N	G	U	Q	G	U	R	B	R
N	X	J	T	F	C	F	B	Q	N	S	J	U	I	P	A	R	P
H	V	A	F	A	A	Z	Z	A	I	U	D	V	A	C	C	A	V
X	S	S	Z	O	R	S	R	O	B	E	E	H	C	T	I	E	S
S	D	J	U	F	S	E	N	S	A	N	M	I	L	X	C	D	L
G	K	Q	I	N	X	S	C	C	Z	E	V	L	K	G	Y	A	I
U	C	K	F	D	M	O	K	A	R	K	W	M	M	L	D	N	A
C	M	J	O	O	P	T	E	O	L	A	Z	D	N	H	E	V	R
E	V	M	T	P	G	M	F	P	X	C	B	G	O	O	M	G	E
V	S	I	J	L	H	M	V	R	K	F	S	M	Y	Z	R	E	D
Q	O	E	O	L	F	Q	A	A	Y	Z	P	I	U	P	C	L	I
N	Y	M	V	W	L	S	D	F	B	P	P	L	D	L	F	F	S

CERVICAL	MOTION
CHEMICAL	RANGE
CONTUSIONS	SAFETY
CPR	SIDERAILS
DISC	THORACIC
LACERATION	VERTEBRAE
LUMBAR	

Chapter Eight
Disasters: Preparedness, Hazards, and Prevention

Objectives

After completing this chapter you should be able to
do the following:

1. Define and correctly spell each of the key terms.

2. List at least four guidelines for managing disasters.

3. Name two agencies involved with developing guidelines
    for safety in the workplace.

4. Identify the main difference between OSHA and NIOSH.

5. List the four parts of an effective hazard communication
    safety program.

6. Name at least three types of potential hazards in the
    hospital work environment.

7. List the three parts of an effective safety program.

Key Terms

- disaster
- Occupational Safety and Health Administration

- triage

Chapter Overview

The ability to function competently during a disaster is a skill that, like each of the other skills in the textbook, takes practice and a sincere desire to learn. Disasters can be frightening, not only to the patient, but to the hospital staff as well. As frightened as you may feel, the patient still expects you, the healthcare worker, to know exactly what to do.

Periodic participation in hospital, interagency, and community disaster drills is your responsibility as a competent healthcare worker. Diligently review the hospital's disaster manual on a regular basis. Willingly volunteer to participate in disaster drills. With that self-initiated training, your participation in a disaster will not be disastrous!

Reading Assignment

Read pages 8-1 through 8-10.

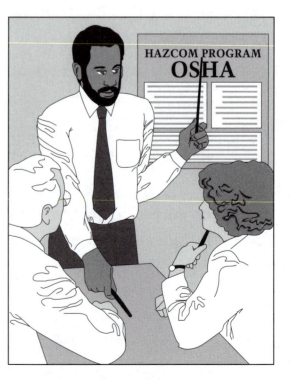

As part of the HazCom program, safety guidelines are designed to protect employees from the dangers of chemicals and medical gases.

Name _____

Date _____

Student Enrichment Activities

Complete the following statements.

1. An unexpected event that causes great damage or exhausts currently available resources is called a _____.

2. A recognized specialty in many departments and agencies concerned with public safety is _____ _____.

3. One of the more common disasters in a hospital occurs from the mishandling of _____ and _____ waste.

4. _____ is responsible for the development and enforcement of job safety and health regulations.

5. Requests submitted by employers or employees concerning working conditions and how they relate to illnesses and diseases contracted by employees are investigated by _____.

6. The key to safety in the workplace is _____.

7. The four parts of the HazCom program are: employee _____, the _____ program, _____ _____ Data Sheets, and _____ _____.

8. An _____ employee is a _____ employee.

Unscramble the following terms.

9. STARSIDE   _____

10. IGREAT   _____

11. STABESOS   _____

12. UNTALCOPAOCI FEYATS   _____ _____

13. ONITALAN ISNUTETIT   _____ _____

Name _____

Date _____

Additional Enrichment Activities

Circle the correct answer.

14. Development and enforcement of job safety and health regulations are the main responsibilities of:
   A. NIOSH.
   B. OSHA.
   C. EPA.
   D. CLIA.

15. The key to safety in the workplace is:
   A. prevention.
   B. following policies and protocols.
   C. developing a safety program.
   D. education.

16. Triage is best defined as:
   A. setting priorities.
   B. a written disaster plan.
   C. to sort.
   D. both A and B.

17. Information provided by the patient is called:
   A. assessment-based.
   B. objective.
   C. opinion-based.
   D. subjective.

18. Proper disaster preparation requires:

    A. thought.

    B. planning and practice.

    C. foresight.

    D. all of the above.

19. Assuring quality in the work environment is mainly the responsibility of:

    A. NIOSH.

    B. OSHA.

    C. the CDC.

    D. none of the above.

Complete the following exercises.

20. Name each of the four parts of a hazard communication program.

    _____

    _____

    _____

    _____

21. Describe the roles of each of the following organizations.

    A. OSHA: _____

    _____

    _____

    _____

    _____

    B. NIOSH: _____

    _____

    _____

    _____

    _____

Name _____

Date _____

22. Identify the ten safety tips to implement should a fire occur in an acute care facility.

_____

_____

_____

_____

_____

_____

_____

_____

_____

23. Describe the steps you would implement as a healthcare worker to help ensure the safety of patients to the scenario described on page 8-6 of the *Introduction to Clinical Allied Healthcare* textbook.

_____

_____

_____

_____

_____

_____

_____

_____

_____

_____

_____

_____

Name _____

Date _____

Disasters: Preparedness, Hazards, and Prevention—Puzzle 1

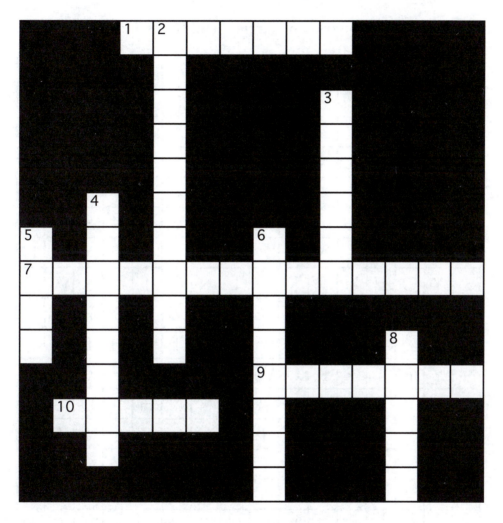

Across

1. Potentially dangerous or deadly conditions existing in a workplace
7. Information provided by a patient about their own condition based on feelings or experience (2 words)
9. Not able to produce children
10. Poisonous

Down

2. An evaluation of a patient's condition
3. To sort or prioritize care for a group of patients
4. A form of magnesium and calcium silicate formerly used in construction and for fireproofing
5. Abbreviation for Occupational Safety and Health Administration
6. An unexpected event that causes great damage and depletes or exhausts currently available resources
8. Abbreviation for National Institute for Occupational Safety and Health

Name _____

Date _____

Disasters: Preparedness, Hazards, and Prevention—Puzzle 2

Find the listed words in the puzzle and circle them. (Contains backwards words.)

D	O	P	S	B	P	F	J	G	M	G	M	H	E	E	N
H	I	S	L	Y	Z	T	D	L	D	P	M	B	W	S	I
A	M	S	H	L	S	X	I	Y	R	A	E	P	F	G	O
Z	P	R	A	A	X	U	Y	O	Y	Z	R	P	H	D	O
A	X	R	X	S	A	D	X	A	E	E	E	Z	N	W	T
R	Y	K	C	O	T	S	O	I	U	V	X	K	S	O	G
D	L	S	R	I	A	E	B	H	G	S	O	T	X	A	U
S	Y	O	H	U	S	K	R	E	N	Q	I	I	S	W	R
K	R	L	F	F	H	F	R	K	S	Z	C	S	P	R	F
J	J	X	O	L	N	L	Y	R	W	T	E	H	E	R	X
M	P	F	I	F	R	U	W	G	T	S	O	F	V	P	K
S	W	F	H	Y	D	X	R	R	S	N	H	S	D	B	M
A	Y	Y	R	M	M	M	I	M	O	O	Z	S	V	F	N
O	W	Y	G	W	F	A	E	E	F	Y	L	Z	O	Q	T
A	X	Y	W	H	G	N	A	U	Y	Z	U	Z	Y	I	U
X	G	M	B	E	T	K	G	H	G	R	N	K	W	B	N

ASBESTOS   NIOSH
ASSESSMENT   OSHA
DISASTER   TOXIC
HAZARDS   TRIAGE

Chapter Nine
Infection Control

Objectives

After completing this chapter you should be able to
do the following:

1. Define and correctly spell each of the key terms.

2. Describe the six components of the infection cycle, and the methods of interrupting each.

3. Thoroughly explain the meaning of the phrase *sterile technique.*

4. List the precautions for preventing puncture wounds from needles and other sharp objects.

5. Explain and demonstrate the proper procedure for donning sterile gloves.

6. Name three serious illnesses clinical health personnel may contract from patients.

7. Describe the main difference between viruses and bacteria.

8. Explain the procedure for proper handwashing.

9. Identify body secretions for which Standard Precautions or Airborne, Droplet, or Contact Precautions must be used.

10. Name the recommended cleaning solution for use in hospitals.

Key Terms

- AIDS
- airborne transmission
- aseptic
- asymptomatic
- bacteria
- Centers for Disease Control and Prevention
- clean technique
- contact transmission
- droplet transmission
- hepatitis A

- hepatitis B
- hepatitis C
- infection cycle
- nosocomial infection
- pathogen
- reverse isolation
- Standard Precautions
- sterile technique
- Transmission-based Precautions
- virus

Chapter Overview

Providing an atmosphere for optimal healing and wellness for the patient is the responsibility of all healthcare workers. This chapter provides insight into the origin of disease (the infection cycle) and proper precautions as set forth by the Centers for Disease Control and Prevention.

The most effective method for reducing the risk of transmitting pathogens between patients is thorough, frequent, and proper handwashing. When providing care for a patient, remember, it is the body secretions that are infectious, not the patient! Never forget, the patient is a person and, therefore, needs personalized care.

Recently, the Centers for Disease Control and Prevention introduced changes for what used to be called *universal precautions* and *body substance isolation*. You must completely understand the new terms and their implications for patient care. Knowing the requirements for donning gloves and other personal protection equipment (PPE) is the main responsibility of the healthcare worker. Practice the proper procedures for donning this equipment and familiarize yourself with the guidelines for wearing the PPE provided by your facility.

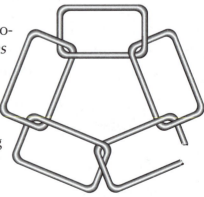

It is important for you to be able to identify the various parts of the infection cycle and take the proper steps to interrupt it.

Reading Assignment

Read pages 9-1 through 9-27.

Name _____

Date _____

Student Enrichment Activities

Complete the following statements.

1. The _____ _____ _____ _____ _____
    _____ is the government agency responsible for protecting the public
    health through the prevention and control of disease.

2. Label the six parts of the infection cycle.

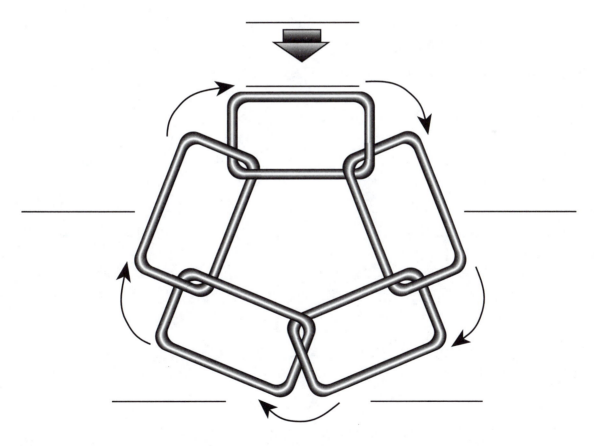

3. Bacteria that need oxygen to grow and reproduce are called _____.

4. *Staph* is an abbreviation for _____.

5. The first step in asepsis is proper and thorough _____.

6. List six times at which handwashing is a MUST. _____

     _____

     _____

7. The preferred method of sterilization is to use an _____ because it destroys all _____.

8. Round bacteria are called _____.

9. Organisms that cause disease are called _____.

10. Bacteria that naturally occurs on various parts of the body are called

     _____.

11. Sterile technique is a precise skill used by _____ _____ who are performing a sterile procedure or assisting with one.

12. The puncture resistant container used for the disposal of needles is called a

     _____ _____.

13. Two diseases that healthcare workers are at risk of contracting are

     _____ and _____.

14. Patients with AIDS are susceptible to _____

     _____.

15. The Centers for Disease Control and Prevention recommend healthcare workers practice the use of _____ _____ if they may be exposed to body fluids.

Name _____

Date _____

16. In hospitals, the recommended cleaning solution is _____ _____

_____.

17. Containment of pathogens to the patient care unit is called _____.

Unscramble the following terms.

18. SAID _____

19. TRACIBEA _____

20. COMSONLOIA _____

21. SETIERL CHQTIENUE _____ _____

22. SPASISE _____

23. IENFITCON CEYLC _____ _____

24. GRAMOCIRMSION _____

25. SIRVU _____

26. SPEITHIAT _____

27. ATROOPZO _____

Name _____

Date _____

Additional Enrichment Activities

Circle the correct answer.

28. The key to medical asepsis is:

    A. autoclaving.

    B. disinfecting patient care items.

    C. using single patient use items only.

    D. proper handwashing.

29. A pathogen is best described as:

    A. a bacterium.

    B. a disease-causing microorganism.

    C. a fungus.

    D. a virus.

30. The Infection Control Department of the hospital is responsible for:

    A. identifying nosocomial infections.

    B. identifying industrial illnesses.

    C. writing and implementing hospital policies and procedures designed to decrease the risk of industrial illness and nosocomial infection.

    D. communicating with the Centers for Disease Control and Prevention.

31. Common portals of entry for various microorganisms include:

    A. breaks in the skin.

    B. the ears.

    C. the mouth and nose.

    D. all of the above.

32. The type of pathogen that gets its food and nutrients from the cell in which it is living is a:

    A. bacterium.

    B. mold.

    C. protozoan.

    D. virus.

33. Bacteria that can grow without O_2 are called:

    A. anaerobic.

    B. streptococci.

    C. aerobic.

    D. staphylococcus.

34. The following are proper steps for correct handwashing EXCEPT:

    A. Always wet your hand with the fingertips pointing down.

    B. Vigorous scrubbing should occur for at least two minutes.

    C. Turn the faucet off using a wet paper towel.

    D. Leave the sink and surrounding area clean and dry.

35. The CDC recommends using _____ solution to disinfect various hospital items.

    A. 10% bleach

    B. 1% bleach

    C. 50% bleach

    D. alcohol

36. The sterile field is considered contaminated:

    A. $1/2$ - 1 inch around the edge.

    B. 1 - $1^1/2$ inch around the edge.

    C. 2 inches around the edge.

    D. There is no area of contamination since all items have been sterilized.

Name _____

Date _____

37. You must thoroughly dry your hands after washing and before donning sterile gloves:

   A. because water can seep through the gloves and cause contamination.

   B. because it allows gloves to be more easily donned.

   C. because moisture permits the growth of bacteria.

   D. It makes no difference if hands are thoroughly dried or moist.

38. Most needle sticks occur because of:

   A. laziness.

   B. battery.

   C. negligence.

   D. written policies and procedures.

39. Standard Precautions and airborne precautions are to be used together for:

   A. the mumps.

   B. varicella.

   C. the common cold.

   D. gastroenteritis.

40. An example of direct patient contact which may result in disease transmission is:

   A. changing the patient's bed linen.

   B. emptying the bedpan or bedside commode.

   C. turning a patient.

   D. none of these.

41. Airborne transmission refers to pathogens that are between:

   A. 0 - 5 microns in size.

   B. 5 - 10 microns in size.

   C. 15 - 20 microns in size.

   D. It refers to pathogens of any size.

42. An example of a disease transmitted by droplets and which requires healthcare workers to don regular masks is:

   A. pneumonia.

   B. pharyngitis.

   C. influenza.

   D. all of these.

43. The measles is transmitted by:

   A. droplets.

   B. droplet nuclei.

   C. blood and blood products.

   D. direct contact.

Complete the following exercises.

44. Describe each of the six links in the cycle of infection.

   _____

   _____

   _____

   _____

   _____

   _____

45. List at least two diseases that may occur through each of the following portals of entry.

   A. skin: _____

   _____

   B. blood and vascular system: _____

   _____

   C. respiratory system: _____

   _____

   D. reproductive and urinary systems: _____

   _____

Name _____

Date _____

46. List the body secretions identified by the Centers for Disease Control and Prevention as possible reservoirs for pathogens.

_____

_____

_____

_____

47. Describe the mode of transmission and causative pathogen for hepatitis A, hepatitis B, and hepatitis C.

_____

_____

_____

_____

_____

_____

48. Describe the steps for each of the following procedures.

A. handwashing: _____

_____

_____

_____

_____

_____

_____

_____

_____

_____

_____

B. donning sterile gloves:_____

_____

_____

_____

_____

_____

_____

_____

_____

_____

_____

_____

_____

_____

_____

_____

_____

_____

_____

_____

C. removing contaminated gloves: _____

_____

_____

_____

_____

_____

_____

_____

_____

_____

_____

Name _____

Date _____

49. Identify how to interrupt the cycle of infection for each link in the chain.

_____

_____

_____

_____

_____

_____

_____

_____

_____

_____

50. Describe and discuss each of the following.

   A. virus: _____

   _____

   _____

   B. bacteria: _____

   _____

   _____

   C. fungi: _____

   _____

   _____

   D. protozoan:_____

   _____

   _____

51. List the indications for use, examples of diseases, and the instructions for healthcare workers for each of the following:

    A. Standard Precautions: _____

    _____

    _____

    B. airborne precautions:_____

    _____

    _____

    _____

    C. droplet precautions: _____

    _____

    _____

    _____

    D. contact precautions: _____

    _____

    _____

    _____

    _____

52. Describe the potential impact of HIV positive and AIDS patients on the medical profession over the next five years, if current trends continue as expected.

    _____

    _____

    _____

    _____

    _____

    _____

    _____

    _____

Name _____

Date _____

Infection Control—Puzzle 1

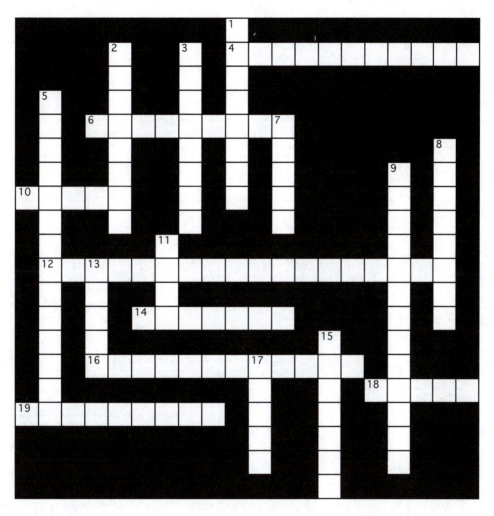

Across

4. Drugs with the ability to kill or prevent the growth of living organisms such as bacteria
6. Disease-causing microorganisms
10. A microscopic, parasitic organism capable of causing an infectious disease
12. See 5 Down (2 words)
14. A condition in which no pathogens, infection, or any form of life is present
16. A body system composed of different types of blood cells that fight off infections (2 words)
18. A liquid; See 3 Down
19. Inflammation of the liver

Down

1. Small, single-celled microorganisms
2. A living thing composed of one or more cells
3. The clear liquid surrounding a joint; with 18 Across
5. A disease caused by HIV that destroys the immune system; with 12 Across (2 words)
7. Abbreviation for the bacteria staphylococcus
8. Those who can spread a disease without showing any outward signs of the disease
9. The liquid contained inside the amnion (2 words)
11. Acquired Immune Deficiency Syndrome
13. Simple parasitic plants such as molds and yeasts
15. Requiring oxygen
17. A type of fungi which may cause disease

Name _____

Date _____

Infection Control—Puzzle 2

Find the listed words in the puzzle and circle them. (Contains backwards words.)

N	K	A	R	T	D	A	H	V	R	C	T	M	E	V	D	B	E
O	E	N	I	P	K	G	Q	K	N	Y	A	Q	I	I	A	W	Y
S	P	L	H	D	Q	C	R	B	D	A	T	R	U	C	Y	L	X
O	H	A	C	P	S	D	D	C	F	G	U	L	T	A	G	G	P
C	O	B	K	Y	A	M	S	W	W	S	F	E	X	F	F	E	A
O	O	V	S	L	C	T	E	W	M	C	R	J	D	T	F	S	Z
M	U	X	J	G	K	N	S	Y	I	I	N	L	F	H	R	N	S
I	R	T	F	R	U	P	O	T	A	N	T	A	G	X	J	E	I
A	C	R	W	E	E	X	O	I	C	S	T	Q	X	U	U	G	T
L	X	G	P	A	F	I	D	Y	T	I	R	M	X	O	K	O	I
I	O	L	W	U	N	S	E	J	U	C	B	E	H	D	V	H	T
D	T	A	H	M	I	A	J	H	F	W	E	O	I	M	N	T	A
Q	G	V	A	S	G	Z	C	L	L	W	S	F	R	R	K	A	P
Y	D	E	P	Y	Y	U	J	N	J	Q	A	J	N	E	R	P	E
P	A	E	K	X	Z	Q	D	F	C	I	G	G	T	I	A	A	H
E	S	J	B	X	H	G	N	O	I	T	A	L	O	S	I	N	C
A	I	M	M	U	N	E	S	Y	S	T	E	M	Y	W	T	U	A
U	R	F	V	G	D	I	U	L	F	L	A	I	V	O	N	Y	S

AIDS	INFECTION CYCLE
AMNIOTIC FLUID	ISOLATION
ANAEROBIC	NOSOCOMIAL
ASEPSIS	PATHOGENS
BACTERIA	STAPH
CARRIERS	SYNOVIAL FLUID
HEPATITIS	VIRUS
IMMUNE SYSTEM	

Chapter Ten
Fundamental Skills

Objectives

After completing this chapter you should be able to
do the following:

1.   Define and correctly spell each of the key terms.

2.   List the four basic vital signs.

3.   Explain three methods of heat loss.

4.   Describe the two different temperature scales.

5.   Explain the term *core temperature.*

6.   Explain the differences between an oral glass thermometer
     and a rectal glass thermometer.

7.   Name the normal numeric value for oral, rectal, and
     axillary temperatures.

8.   Identify five locations on the body where a pulse can be felt.

9.   Describe the normal resting heart rate for an adult.

10.   Identify at least three conditions that can change a heart rate.

11.   Describe the respiratory cycle.

12.   Explain the term *blood pressure.*

Key Terms

- artery
- blood pressure
- bradycardia
- Celsius
- central circulation
- core temperature
- diaphragm
- diastolic
- Fahrenheit
- homeostasis
- hypertension

- hypothalamus
- peripheral circulation
- PMI
- pulse
- respiration
- systolic
- tachycardia
- trauma
- vein
- vital signs

Chapter Overview

You are now approximately halfway through the text. Chapter Ten introduces you to fundamental skills for patient care. It will be your responsibility to practice each skill properly and to understand the reason presented for each step.

DO NOT try to shortcut any of the steps to these procedures! Only when you have more experience will you be able to give medically sound reasons for changing the sequence of steps in performing a skill. This chapter requires PRACTICE, which will demand self-initiative on YOUR part.

Enjoy learning each of these skills, and try to understand their importance to your career in the medical profession.

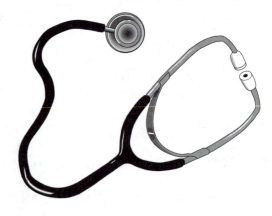

Reading Assignment

Read pages 10-1 through 10-45.

It is important for you to be able to obtain accurate measurements for each of the vital signs.

Name _____

Date _____

Student Enrichment Activities

Complete the following statements.

1. _____ _____ provide the healthcare worker with
    information concerning the health status of the body.

2. _____, _____, and _____ are
    methods of heat loss.

3. The maintenance of equilibrium within the body through internal and external
    functions is called _____.

4. The oral or rectal methods are preferred for measurements of the _____
    _____.

5. The _____ temperature registers approximately 1° higher than the
    oral temperature.

6. The rhythmic throbbing caused by the regular contraction and expansion of an
    artery is the _____.

7. The blood flow supplied to the vital organs is the _____ circulation.

8. Gas exchange involves exchanging _____ _____ for
    _____.

9. The temporary cessation of breathing is _____.

10. A sphygmomanometer is used in taking a _____ blood
    pressure reading.

11. When charting the weight of an adult patient, pounds should be converted to

_____.

12. Write this Fahrenheit thermometer reading in the blank below.

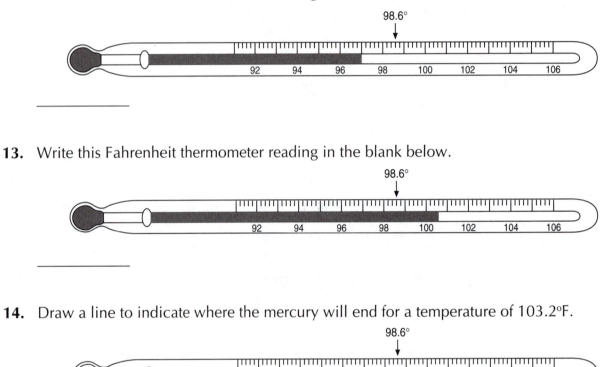

_____

13. Write this Fahrenheit thermometer reading in the blank below.

_____

14. Draw a line to indicate where the mercury will end for a temperature of 103.2°F.

15. Write this Celsius thermometer reading in the blank below.

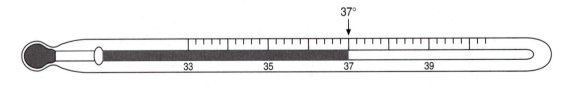

_____

16. Write this Celsius thermometer reading in the blank below.

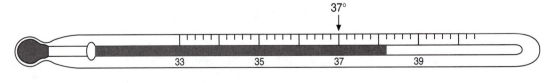

_____

Name _____

Date _____

17. Draw a line to indicate where the mercury will end for a temperature of 39.4°C.

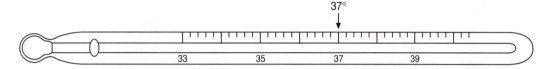

Write the sphygmomanometer readings in the spaces below.

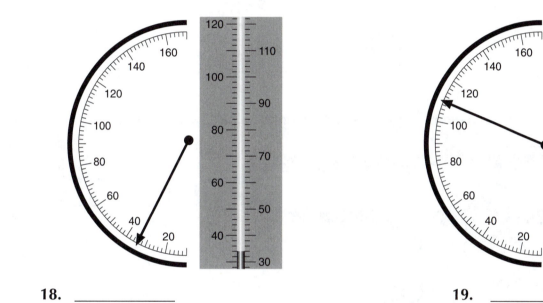

18. _____

19. _____

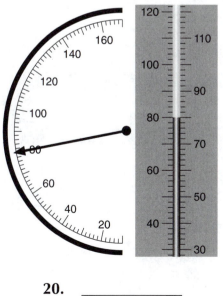

20. _____

Write the height measurements in the spaces below.

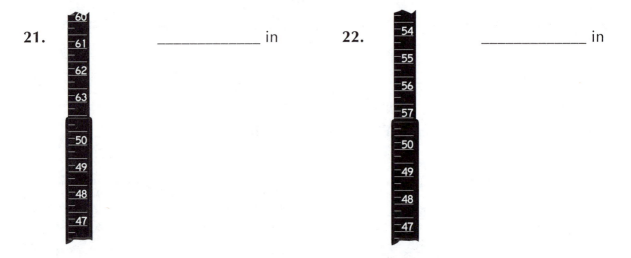

21. _____ in   22. _____ in

Write the weight measurements in pounds and kilograms in the spaces below.

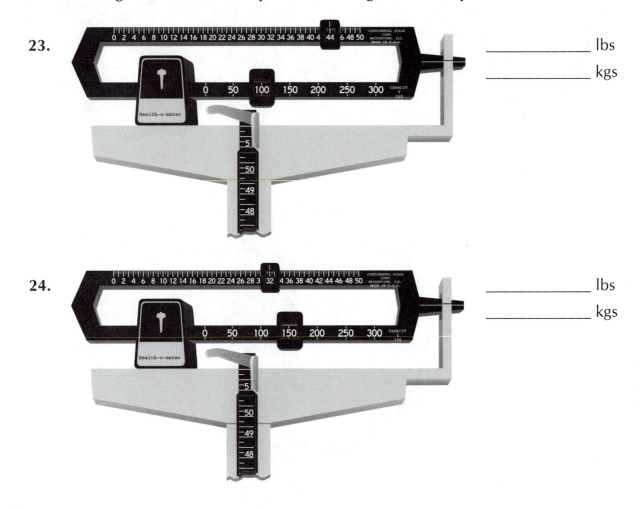

23. _____ lbs
    _____ kgs

24. _____ lbs
    _____ kgs

Name _____

Date _____

Unscramble the following terms.

25. PEAX   _____

26. ROADTIC   _____

27. AGS ECXNGHAE   _____ _____

28. TRIADANIO   _____

29. SUMALSKUS   _____

30. ERSIOPATIRN   _____

31. SCHOOPTESTE   _____

32. PYATHECAN   _____

33. RYDEATH   _____

34. NEVI   _____

35. YCNEHE KSOTSE   _____ _____

Name _____

Date _____

Additional Enrichment Activities

Circle the correct answer.

36. Homeostasis refers to:

    A. a chemical process by which heat is produced.

    B. a portion of the brain that controls the temperature of the body.

    C. an assessment process of the body functions essential to life.

    D. a state of equilibrium within the body that is maintained through adaptation of the body systems.

37. Blood pressure, temperature, pulse, and respirations:

    A. are called vital signs.

    B. provide essential information concerning the condition of the body.

    C. are indicators of Kussmaul's triad.

    D. both A and B.

38. Apnea is:

    A. the temporary cessation of spontaneous breathing.

    B. a respiratory rate below 12 breaths per minute.

    C. a respiratory rate above 24 breaths per minute.

    D. none of the above.

39. To convert a patient's weight from pounds to kilograms, you must:

    A. multiply the number of pounds by 2.2.

    B. divide the number of pounds by $5/9$.

    C. divide the number of pounds by 2.2.

    D. multiply the number of pounds by $5/9$.

40. Tachypnea refers to:

    A. an abnormally rapid respiratory rate.

    B. an abnormally rapid cardiac rate.

    C. an abnormally slow respiratory rate.

    D. an abnormally slow cardiac rate.

41. Stridor is:

    A. another name for sphygmomanometer.

    B. a high-pitched respiratory sound due to upper airway obstruction.

    C. a high-pitched respiratory sound due to lower airway obstruction.

    D. an unstable gait.

42. Tachycardia refers to:

    A. an abnormally rapid respiratory rate.

    B. an abnormally low cardiac rate.

    C. an abnormally high respiratory rate.

    D. an abnormally high cardiac rate.

43. To convert a patient's temperature from Fahrenheit to Celsius:

    A. subtract 32 from the Fahrenheit value and multiply by $9/5$.

    B. multiply the Fahrenheit value by $9/5$ and add 32.

    C. subtract 32 from the Fahrenheit value and multiply by $5/9$.

    D. multiply the Fahrenheit value by $5/9$ and add 32.

44. A tympanic temperature is obtained:

    A. by placing a thermometer strip on the forehead.

    B. by placing the thermometer over the opening to the external auditory canal.

    C. by placing the thermometer under the tongue.

    D. by placing the thermometer in the axilla.

Name _____

Date _____

45. The core temperature may be affected by:

    A. CVAs.

    B. body fat.

    C. the time of day.

    D. all of the above.

46. The pulse rate may be affected by:

    A. medications.

    B. hyperpyrexia.

    C. emotions.

    D. all of the above.

47. The name of the pulse located next to the trachea is the:

    A. carotid pulse.

    B. common pulse.

    C. central pulse.

    D. cardiac pulse.

48. The pulse most commonly used to assess peripheral circulation is the:

    A. carotid pulse.

    B. pedal pulse.

    C. radial pulse.

    D. femoral pulse.

49. The correct location for obtaining the apical pulse is:

    A. the third intercostal space, left anterior chest.

    B. the fifth intercostal space, left posterior chest, inferior to the left scapula.

    C. the third intercostal space, left anterior chest, inferior to the left nipple.

    D. the fifth intercostal space, left anterior chest, inferior to the left nipple.

50. Inhalation occurs when:

    A. the level of O_2 declines below normal.

    B. the level of CO_2 increases above normal.

    C. the levels of O_2 and CO_2 become even with each other.

    D. the level of CO_2 declines below normal.

51. Crackles indicate fluid in the:

    A. pulmonary vein.

    B. pulmonary artery.

    C. bronchial tubes.

    D. alveoli.

52. The common measurements obtained for blood pressure are:

    A. diaphragm.

    B. diastolic.

    C. systolic.

    D. both B and C.

53. When obtaining a palpated blood pressure, the measurement omitted is:

    A. pulse pressure.

    B. diaphragm.

    C. diastolic.

    D. systolic.

Name _____

Date _____

Complete the following exercises.

54. Describe the proper procedure for obtaining a palpated blood pressure.

_____

_____

_____

_____

_____

_____

_____

_____

_____

_____

_____

_____

_____

_____

_____

55. Describe the difference or differences between central circulation and peripheral circulation.

_____

_____

_____

_____

_____

56. Write down each step, in the proper order, for obtaining a radial pulse. Which circulation does this pulse assess and why?

_____

_____

_____

_____

_____

_____

_____

_____

_____

_____

_____

57. List the guidelines for determining the normal heart rates for the following:

A. infants: _____

_____

B. children (1-7 years old): _____

_____

C. children (over 7 years old): _____

_____

D. adults: _____

_____

58. List the pulse sites used to assess peripheral circulation.

_____

_____

_____

Name _____

Date _____

59. Describe three methods of heat loss.

_____

_____

_____

_____

_____

_____

60. List the types of conditions that may affect the following vital signs.

A. pulse: _____

_____

B. temperature: _____

_____

C. respiratory rate: _____

_____

D. blood pressure: _____

_____

61. Thoroughly define each of the following terms.

A. dyspnea: _____

_____

B. tachypnea: _____

_____

C. Kussmaul's respiration: _____

_____

D. hypertension: _____

_____

E. systolic: _____

_____

F. diastolic: _____

_____

G. homeostasis: _____

_____

H. vital signs: _____

_____

I. core temperature: _____

_____

J. peripheral circulation: _____

_____

K. central circulation: _____

_____

L. tachycardia: _____

_____

M. bradycardia: _____

_____

Name _____

Date _____

Fundamental Skills—Puzzle 1

Across

8. The eardrum (2 words)
11. Examine by feeling with the hands
12. The temporary cessation of spontaneous breathing
14. Lying on one side with the arms and legs drawn toward the chest and the head bowed (2 words)
17. The pulse found on the inside of the arm near the elbow
18. A metric fluid measurement equal to 1000 milliliters
19. Bringing oxygen into the body and expelling carbon dioxide
20. Grossly irregular breathing

Down

1. High blood pressure based on several random readings of 140/90 or higher
2. A breathing pattern with deep, gasping respirations; "air hunger"
3. Abnormally rapid breathing
4. The bottom number in a blood pressure reading
5. The pointed tip of the heart
6. The temperature scale that uses 212° as the boiling point of water and 32° as the freezing point of water
7. The pulse found in the groin area
9. The pulse located on both sides of the neck next to the trachea
10. Physical or psychological injury
13. A blood vessel that carries low-oxygenated blood to the heart
15. A quantitative measurement of the heartbeat
16. A blood vessel that carries highly oxygenated blood away from the heart to the tissues

Name _____

Date _____

Fundamental Skills—Puzzle 2

Find the listed words in the puzzle and circle them. (Contains backwards words.)

E	S	A	G	R	K	W	T	K	L	U	A	M	S	S	U	K	A
M	O	P	A	J	C	S	B	F	X	F	F	F	N	G	W	P	J
W	E	E	G	O	D	I	N	J	B	Z	Z	Z	O	U	I	N	V
H	B	R	J	T	Y	J	I	I	K	P	P	I	V	C	U	S	I
P	D	A	A	A	M	D	R	H	U	Y	V	X	A	R	I	I	U
D	A	P	X	S	O	I	N	L	W	C	W	L	L	O	Z	S	S
H	I	L	A	J	V	U	K	L	Z	D	B	A	C	L	E	P	Z
O	B	T	P	J	M	L	B	Z	S	E	R	I	M	C	V	A	K
B	H	R	O	A	Z	B	N	C	C	O	L	F	Z	J	D	B	J
V	K	P	A	R	T	Y	S	Z	M	O	X	P	I	N	H	Q	H
G	N	X	H	C	A	E	V	E	T	R	H	U	P	R	D	L	G
A	T	C	T	O	H	C	F	S	U	J	F	N	B	X	M	V	Z
B	U	W	A	P	M	I	A	T	V	K	F	N	M	T	I	I	D
P	H	U	O	U	M	I	A	I	R	J	J	N	C	V	P	P	A
X	K	N	J	C	D	G	K	L	F	A	S	N	Z	Z	B	W	E
C	R	Q	F	F	T	D	Q	J	Z	H	U	M	Y	O	V	V	N
E	M	D	M	B	V	F	B	Y	T	W	M	M	X	G	L	X	P
F	A	U	W	D	U	A	G	I	A	T	Q	V	A	L	T	U	A

APICAL   FEMORAL
APNEA   KUSSMAUL
BRACHIAL   PALPATE
CAROTID   TRAUMA
DIASTOLIC

Chapter Eleven
Fundamental Patient Care Equipment

Objectives

After completing this chapter you should be able to
do the following:

1. Define and correctly spell each of the key terms.

2. List at least three basic ambulation devices.

3. Describe the universal method for identifying oxygen.

4. Explain the components of a urinary catheter.

5. Explain the procedure for using a patient lift.

6. List at least six items found on the crash cart.

7. Name three reasons why a patient may be in a private room.

8. List five items that can be found in a patient unit.

Key Terms

- activities of daily living
- ambulation
- bedside commode
- call light
- cardiopulmonary arrest
- cardiopulmonary resuscitation (CPR)
- Code Blue
- crash cart
- eggcrate mattress

- gurney
- indwelling catheter
- intercom system
- IV infusion pump
- patient lift
- patient unit
- traction
- wheelchair

Chapter Overview

Chapter Eleven addresses basic patient care equipment. The theme of the textbook has been PATIENTS DESERVE AND EXPECT COMPETENT PATIENT CARE. In other words, patients expect you to know what you are doing. That includes being familiar with patient care equipment and how it works.

Remember to never use a piece of equipment for which you have not been trained. This is not only potentially risky for the patient, but for your safety as well. Most of the equipment in hospitals is extremely costly. Negligence in its use is not acceptable.

As you enter the clinical internship phase of your training, actively seek out the various pieces of equipment. Read their instructions and ask questions of your clinical instructor regarding operation and indications for use. This will serve to increase your clinical knowledge and skills, and make you a more valuable employee.

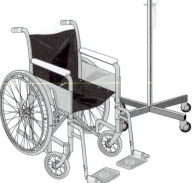

Reading Assignment

Read pages 11-1 through 11-15.

Give your patients the best care possible by learning the proper way to use equipment.

Name _____

Date _____

Student Enrichment Activities

Complete the following statements.

1. The word _____ refers to the process of walking.

2. Three examples of commonly used ambulation devices are _____,
   _____ , and _____.

3. An eggcrate mattress helps prevent skin _____.

4. The universal color indicating oxygen is _____.

5. Most intravenous solutions are administered through an _____
   _____ pump.

6. A tube that is inserted to drain the urinary bladder is an _____
   _____.

7. A _____ _____ is a specially-equipped cart used for
   cardiopulmonary arrests.

8. An _____ _____ is often used to apply heat therapy
   to a patient.

9. Patients with an extremely low body temperature are often placed on a
   _____ _____.

10. A patient communication device contained within the patient care unit is the
    intercom and _____ _____ system.

Unscramble the following terms.

11. LAMBTAUNIO   _____

12. RCSAH TCRA   _____   _____

13. LINGLINDEW THEATERC   _____   _____

14. TSKRYER EARFM   _____   _____

15. CLEAHWERHI   _____

16. DBE CELDAR   _____   _____

17. PLAYDARIONCRUOM STARRE   _____   _____

18. RUNGEY   _____

19. SLIEBURZEN   _____

20. ICONRATT   _____

21. ECDO ULEB   _____   _____

22. DEISBDE MOEMDOC   _____   _____

23. TEPANIT FLIT   _____   _____

24. LASAN CANLANU   _____   _____

Name _____

Date _____

Additional Enrichment Activities

Circle the correct answer.

25. Examples of excretory equipment include:

   A. indwelling catheters.

   B. suctioning equipment.

   C. incentive spirometers.

   D. both A and B.

26. The special bed used for patients with full-body burns or spinal cord injuries is:

   A. a Stryker frame.

   B. a patient lift.

   C. a gurney.

   D. a bed scale.

27. The purpose of traction is to:

   A. reduce pain.

   B. allow body movement around the immobilized body part.

   C. stop bleeding.

   D. properly align the body part to promote healing.

28. *Code Blue* means:

   A. a fire.

   B. a hazardous material incident.

   C. a cardiopulmonary arrest.

   D. all of the above.

29. A crash cart is equipped with:

    A. an O_2 tank.

    B. cardiac medications.

    C. a suction apparatus.

    D. all of the above.

Complete the following exercises.

30. List the items that may be contained in the patient care unit.

_____

_____

_____

_____

31. Identify three types of ambulation devices, describe how the devices operate, and explain why each may be used.

_____

_____

_____

_____

_____

_____

_____

_____

_____

_____

_____

Name _____

Date _____

32. List at least four respiratory devices and explain when each may be used.

_____

_____

_____

_____

_____

_____

_____

_____

_____

_____

_____

_____

_____

_____

33. List the equipment that may be included on a crash cart.

_____

_____

_____

_____

_____

34. Explain how each of the following devices function.

A. Roto-Rest bed: _____

_____

_____

B. alternating pressure mattress: _____

_____

_____

C. eggcrate mattress:_____

_____

_____

D. Stryker frame: _____

_____

_____

35. List four reasons why a patient may be admitted to a private patient care unit.

_____

_____

_____

_____

_____

_____

_____

Name _____

Date _____

Fundamental Patient Care Equipment—Puzzle 1

Across

4. A bag connected to an indwelling catheter to collect body fluids (2 words)
5. A portable supply cabinet that contains emergency equipment for a full arrest (2 words)
8. A combination of water, dextrose, and other electrolytes that replenishes essential nutrients (2 words)
11. Bedding made of foam which is used to prevent skin breakdown (2 words)
14. Cardiopulmonary resuscitation
15. Provides dry heat via heated water that is electrically circulated (2 words)
16. A special chair equipped with wheels for transporting patients

Down

1. Refers to pulse and respirations
2. Delivers a fine spray or mist of medication
3. Pulling a part of the body into proper alignment
5. Used by patients to call the nurses' station (2 words)
6. The process of walking
7. A bed used to change a patient's position to relieve constant pressure (2 words)
9. A special oxygen tube that is placed just inside each nostril (2 words)
10. An ambulation assistance device (comes with or without wheels)
12. The emergency call signal for a full arrest (2 words)
13. To bring to a stop; often used with 1 Down

Name _____

Date _____

Fundamental Patient Care Equipment—Puzzle 2

Find the listed words in the puzzle and circle them. (Contains backwards words.)

C	I	S	T	R	Q	S	R	O	T	A	L	I	T	N	E	V	D
R	O	V	E	Z	K	P	X	X	R	F	X	D	W	A	Y	A	J
Y	J	D	F	D	T	U	C	S	L	Y	N	O	L	E	P	R	T
A	D	W	E	L	O	D	C	H	J	A	M	U	N	K	J	C	O
B	H	D	X	B	U	M	I	F	N	O	N	R	A	W	D	V	Y
I	C	C	H	U	L	I	M	D	S	N	U	U	P	Q	E	X	H
N	U	Z	X	Z	I	U	D	O	A	G	Q	P	J	P	P	W	R
O	M	W	D	L	N	P	E	C	C	A	T	C	N	V	P	Y	I
I	Y	N	J	S	Z	V	L	C	C	E	V	Z	Z	R	F	O	A
T	N	C	Q	V	L	A	A	U	S	R	D	R	V	S	I	D	H
A	V	O	D	R	S	L	N	S	H	D	A	I	L	V	K	U	C
L	Q	E	F	A	L	O	H	P	U	H	T	S	S	T	T	C	L
U	G	F	N	L	I	R	Y	C	R	U	B	N	H	D	Z	O	E
B	W	W	I	T	R	U	O	S	V	M	A	O	K	C	E	I	E
M	M	G	C	C	Q	C	F	N	Q	L	P	L	C	D	A	B	H
A	H	A	V	M	O	J	J	O	V	P	S	L	K	O	R	R	W
T	R	V	T	W	V	G	C	T	Q	Z	L	C	T	Q	H	P	T
T	J	D	M	Y	E	M	A	R	F	R	E	K	Y	R	T	S	C

AMBULATION   GURNEY

AQUA-K PAD   IV FLUID

BEDSIDE COMMODE   NASAL CANNULA

CALL LIGHT   STRYKER FRAME

CODE BLUE   TRACTION

CPR   VENTILATORS

CRASH CART   WHEELCHAIR

Chapter Twelve
Introduction to Medical Terminology

Objectives

After completing this chapter you should be able to
do the following:

1. Define and correctly spell each of the key terms.

2. Correctly spell, define, and use all of the medical abbreviations.

3. Identify prefixes, suffixes, and combining forms from selected medical terms.

4. Identify medical abbreviations from a selected list.

Key Terms

- combining form
- combining vowel
- prefix

- root word
- suffix

Chapter Overview

Medicine has its own terminology and approved abbreviations. As a competent healthcare worker, you must not only walk the walk, but you must also CORRECTLY talk the talk.

Chapter Twelve provides the backbone for proper communication and documentation in the medical profession. It requires an immense amount of memorization, and only YOU can do that. Complete all of the exercises and practice what you are learning.

Reading Assignment

Read pages 12-1 through 12-21.

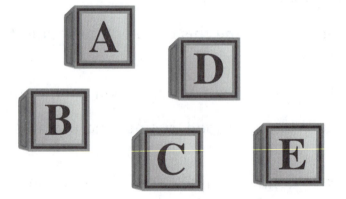

Your ability to provide quality patient care requires mastery of the basic building blocks for medical terminology.

Name _____

Date _____

Student Enrichment Activities

Define the following prefixes, roots (combining forms), and suffixes.

1. arteri/o: _____ .

2. -algia: _____ .

3. anti-: _____ .

4. arthr/o: _____ .

5. audi/o: _____ .

6. cephal/o: _____ .

7. chol/o: _____ .

8. derm/o: _____ .

9. cyan/o: _____ .

10. circum-: _____ .

11. cyst/o: _____ .

12. dys-: _____ .

13. epi-: _____ .

14. -ectomy: _____ .

15. glyc/o: _____ .

16. -gram: _____ .

17. enter/o: _____ .

18. gynec/o: _____ .

19. hydr/o: _____ .

20. hepat/o: _____ .

21. intra-: _____ .

22. -itis: _____ .

23. lip/o: _____ .

24. -logy: _____ .

25. mal-: _____ .

26. nephr/o: _____ .

27. oste/o: _____ . 29. -tomy:_____ .

28. -stomy: _____ . 30. peri-:_____ .

Define the following.

31. cholecystectomy: _____ .

32. dysuria: _____ .

33. glycosuria:_____ .

34. hepatitis: _____ .

35. hydrocephalus: _____ .

36. hysterectomy: _____ .

37. appendicitis: _____ .

38. lipase:_____ .

39. ABGs:_____ .

40. AMI: _____ .

41. BCP: _____ .

42. BP: _____ .

43. BUE: _____ .

Name _____

Date _____

44. epicardial: _____ .

45. pericarditis: _____ .

46. gynecology: _____ .

47. arteriogram: _____ .

48. nephritis: _____ .

49. CNS: _____ .

50. DAT: _____ .

51. pleuritis: _____ .

52. EKG: _____ .

53. FBS: _____ .

54. GI: _____ .

55. gastritis: _____ .

56. AIDS: _____ .

57. dermatitis: _____ .

58. myalgia: _____ .

59. IM: _____ .

60. OTC: _____ .

61. OR: _____ .

62. pathology: _____ .

63. RN: _____ .

64. TPR: _____ .

65. XR: _____ .

66. pleur/o: _____ .

67. -pnea: _____ .

68. path/o: _____ .

69. phleb/o: _____ .

70. pseud/o: _____ .

71. retr/o: _____ .

72. -scopy: _____ .

73. sub-: _____ .

74. supra-: _____ .

Name _____

Date _____

75. thromb/o: _____ .

76. -uria: _____ .

77. vas/o: _____ .

78. viscer/o: _____ .

Unscramble the following terms.

79. DEAMCIL TROMINGLOEY   _____ _____

80. FREXIP   _____

81. FUFSIX   _____

82. MONTIOMUNCIAC   _____

83. NOACTEMDUNTOI   _____

84. CIDARRESITIP   _____

85. TOMASEGRYTC   _____

Name _____

Date _____

Additional Enrichment Activities

Circle the correct answer.

86. Cost/o means:
   A. a fluid-filled sac.
   B. blue.
   C. muscle.
   D. rib.

87. -ase means:
   A. enzyme.
   B. vessel.
   C. against.
   D. side.

88. Dermatology is:
   A. one who studies diseases of the skin.
   B. the study of movement.
   C. the study of the skin.
   D. the study of digits.

89. A histofreezer would be a device that would:
   A. freeze the uterus.
   B. freeze the liver.
   C. freeze blood.
   D. freeze tissue.

90. CC is the abbreviation for:
    A. Critical Care Unit.
    B. chief complaint.
    C. cubic centimeter.
    D. crash cart.

91. In the word *anemia*, the word element *-emia* means:
    A. leukocytes.
    B. blood.
    C. platelets.
    D. lack of.

92. Dysuria means:
    A. difficulty breathing.
    B. painful urination.
    C. difficult or painful flow.
    D. painful breathing.

93. The word element placed in front of the main part of a word is the:
    A. suffix.
    B. root.
    C. prefix.
    D. stem.

94. Inflammation of the covering of the lungs is called:
    A. pericarditis.
    B. pleuritis.
    C. bronchitis.
    D. laryngotracheobronchitis.

Name _____

Date _____

95. KUB is the abbreviation for:

    A. kidney, urethra, bladder.

    B. kidney, ureter, bladder.

    C. kidney, uterus, bladder.

    D. either A or B.

Complete the following exercises.

96. Describe the process for determining the meaning of a medical term.

_____

_____

_____

_____

_____

97. Define the following and give at least three examples of each.

    A. root word: _____

    _____

    B. prefix: _____

    _____

    C. suffix: _____

    _____

    D. combining vowel: _____

    _____

    E. combining form:_____

    _____

Name _____

Date _____

Introduction to Medical Terminology—Puzzle 1

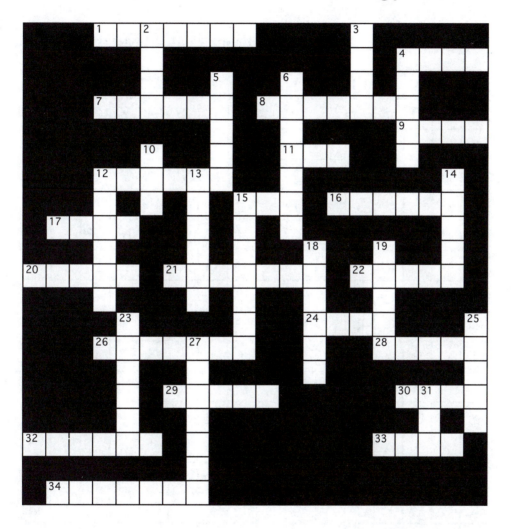

Across

1. Dilation, expansion, or stretching
4. Half or partial
7. Twisted
8. Head
9. Many
11. Upon, over, or upper
12. False
15. Three
16. Excessive flow
17. Record
20. Near
21. Arm
22. White
24. Against
26. Viscera, internal organs
28. Vessel, either blood or lymph
29. Blue
30. Pushing or driving away
32. Surgical removal, excision
33. The ilium, part of hip bone
34. Pertaining to the meninges

Down

2. Order, arrangement, or coordination
3. Enlarged
4. Visual examination
5. Rib
6. Movement
10. Blood
12. Surgical repair
13. Right side
14. Lips
15. Windpipe
18. The body
19. Lack of or deficiency
23. Surrounding or around
25. Alike or the same
27. Red
31. One

Name _____

Date _____

Introduction to Medical Terminology—Puzzle 2

Find the listed words in the puzzle and circle them. (Contains backwards words.)

K	C	W	Z	O	X	D	B	M	T	H	Y	N	V	G	O
X	D	D	M	A	H	R	O	H	P	W	M	Z	G	W	F
X	D	L	I	Y	E	R	R	D	Z	B	P	K	W	O	M
T	U	B	P	C	T	O	L	Z	D	M	B	V	B	M	V
P	A	E	S	S	M	H	R	T	X	M	B	T	A	A	N
L	R	I	A	B	C	J	E	X	V	P	C	N	Z	N	P
J	V	G	O	Z	T	I	P	P	M	W	S	F	D	T	J
Q	O	G	O	H	H	M	S	I	A	G	Z	I	K	O	A
M	B	X	Y	K	N	U	F	C	E	T	O	Y	R	C	D
J	V	R	X	J	E	T	G	T	I	G	J	G	F	W	R
T	N	A	P	Y	N	F	Y	H	X	R	N	U	I	V	L
Y	Y	Q	Z	E	E	K	Z	I	U	J	T	I	X	L	Q
U	R	I	A	M	H	L	Q	V	P	K	S	A	N	T	O
J	N	U	A	A	I	S	N	A	O	P	Y	H	I	E	A
R	S	R	V	Y	A	V	R	P	Y	S	O	T	C	E	M
S	O	M	A	T	L	L	I	T	Q	U	B	A	Q	K	Q

ECTO	MENING
GASTRO	OLIGO
HEPAT	PULMO
HYPER	SOMAT
HYPO	THROMBO
IATRICS	URIA
JUXTA	VISCER
LABIA	

Chapter Thirteen
An Introduction to the Human Body

Objectives

After completing this chapter, you should be able to do the following:

1. Define and correctly spell each of the key terms.

2. Name and explain the function of at least four cellular components.

3. Explain the function of enzymes.

4. Describe two kinds of reproductive processes.

5. Name and describe the four different types of tissue groups.

6. Name the three kinds of muscle tissue.

7. Explain the requirements of a body system.

8. Identify the three directional planes.

9. Name the three sections of the anterior cavity.

10. Name the two sections of the posterior cavity.

11. Identify the body organs that are contained within each of the body cavities.

Key Terms

- anatomy
- cell
- connective tissue
- edema
- epithelial tissue
- meiosis
- mitosis

- muscle tissue
- nerve tissue
- organ
- physiology
- semipermeable
- system

Chapter Overview

Chapter Thirteen provides a firm foundation of information regarding anatomy and physiology, enabling you to provide better healthcare for your patients. You will need to memorize terms, locations, and concepts. Diligent study and frequent repetition will help you master the more difficult concepts.

You are strongly encouraged to complete each of the exercises for this chapter. The information contained within this chapter must be thoroughly understood prior to continuing in the text.

Reading Assignment

Read pages 13-1 through 13-10.

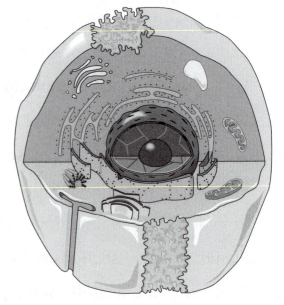

The cell is the most basic unit of life.

Name _____

Date _____

Student Enrichment Activities

Complete the following statements.

1. The jelly-like material contained within a cell is called _____.

2. The _____ is the basis of all living things.

3. The two types of cell division are _____ and _____.

4. The amount of energy released during the chemical reactions that occur in cells is determined by _____.

5. The four types of tissues are _____, _____, _____, and _____.

6. _____ muscle attaches to bones and permits movement.

7. Imaginary lines that separate the body into sections are called _____ _____.

8. The _____, or _____, cavity is the body cavity located along the front part of the body.

Unscramble the following terms.

9. MEADE _____

10. POISADE _____

11. EOSSUOS   _____

12. THLIAPEIEL   _____

13. SVRETRENSA LAPEN   _____   _____

14. GLIATTDISAM LAPNE   _____   _____

15. SODRLA CYTIVA   _____   _____

16. CITRHOAC AVTICY   _____   _____

Name _____

Date _____

Additional Enrichment Activities

Circle the correct answer.

17. Epithelial tissue is the same as:

    A. osseous tissue.

    B. connective tissue.

    C. nerve tissue.

    D. none of the above.

18. Water accounts for about _____ of the body's weight.

    A. 40%

    B. 50%

    C. 60%

    D. 70%

19. Which plane divides the body into right and left halves?

    A. The frontal plane

    B. The coronal plane

    C. The midsagittal plane

    D. The ventral plane

20. The division of human reproductive cells is called:

    A. mitosis.

    B. meiosis.

    C. myelitis.

    D. myofibrosis.

21. The part of the cell responsible for the chemical reactions within the cell is the:
    A. organelle.
    B. nucleolus.
    C. endoplasmic reticulum.
    D. mitochondria.

22. Adipose tissue is a type of:
    A. soft connective tissue.
    B. fibrous connective tissue.
    C. epithelial tissue.
    D. visceral tissue.

23. The human body contains ____ cavities.
    A. 3
    B. 9
    C. 2
    D. 5

24. The medical term that indicates the amount of tissue fluid is:
    A. edema.
    B. tenting.
    C. dehydration.
    D. all of the above.

25. The plane that divides the body into upper and lower halves is called:
    A. the transvertical plane.
    B. the transeptal plane.
    C. the transverse plane.
    D. the translinear plane.

Name _____

Date _____

26. A special feature of the cell membrane is:

    A. nonpermeability.

    B. semipermeability.

    C. homeostasis.

    D. its ability to change composition.

Complete the following exercises.

27. List and describe the three types of muscle tissue.

_____

_____

_____

28. Name each of the body cavities and the organ(s) contained within each.

_____

_____

_____

_____

_____

_____

_____

_____

29. Define the following terms.

A. midsagittal plane: _____

_____

B. coronal plane: _____

_____

C. distal: _____

_____

D. proximal: _____

_____

E. cytoplasm: _____

_____

F. mitochondria: _____

_____

G. meiosis: _____

_____

H. mitosis: _____

_____

I. anatomy: _____

_____

J. physiology: _____

30. List and describe the four main types of tissue groups.

_____

_____

_____

_____

_____

_____

_____

_____

Name _____

Date _____

Fill in the blanks for each of the following diagrams.

31.   The Parts of a Human Cell

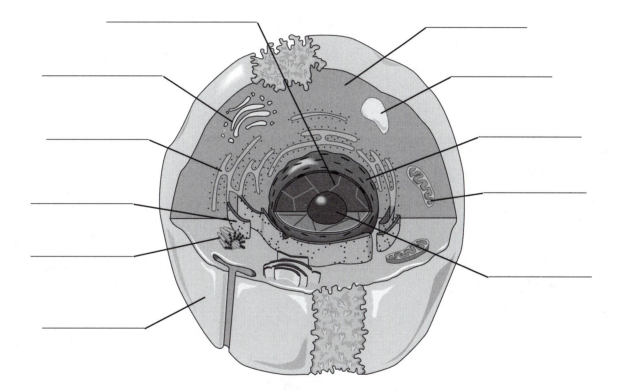

32. From Cell to System

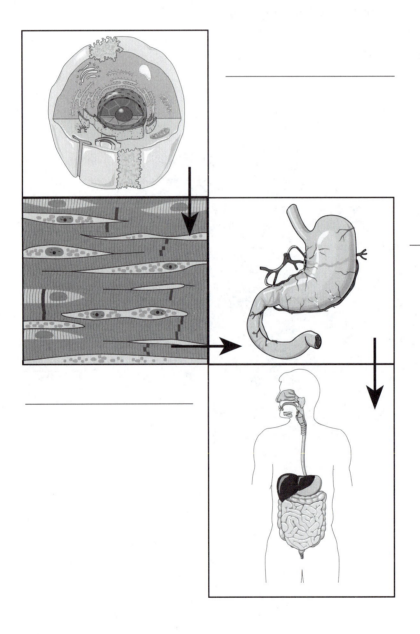

_____

_____

_____

_____

Name _____

Date _____

33. Directional Planes and Terms

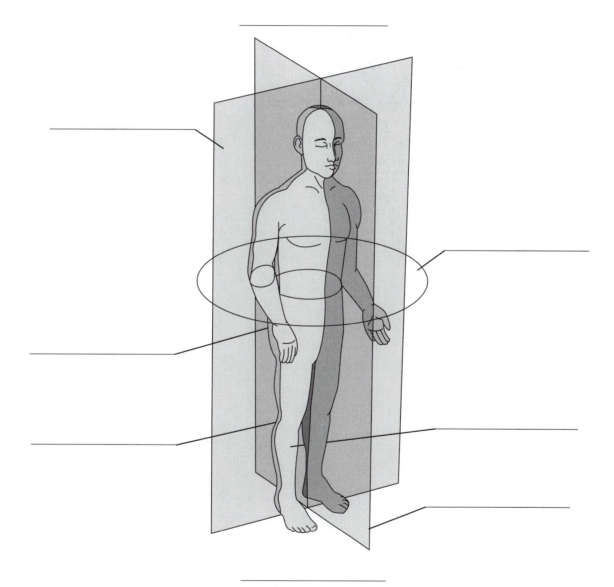

34. The Body Cavities

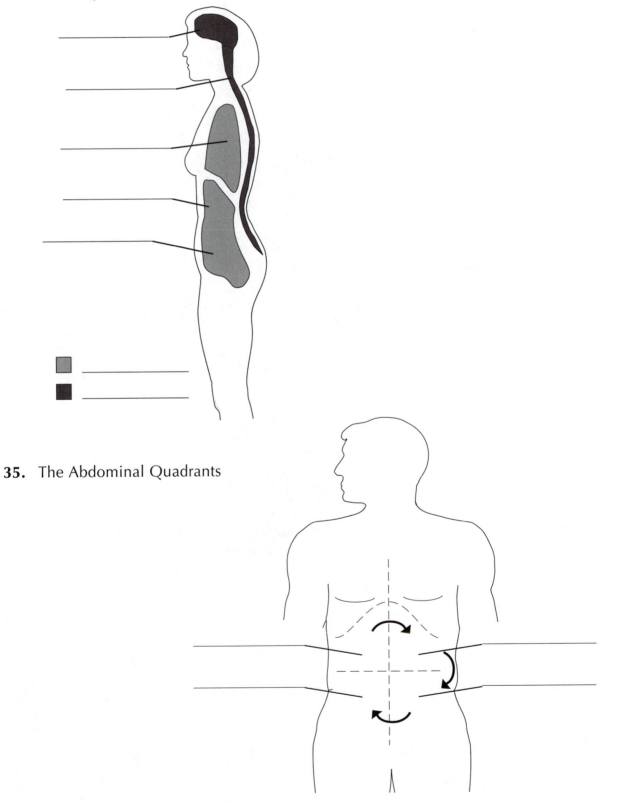

35. The Abdominal Quadrants

Name _____

Date _____

Introduction to the Human Body—Puzzle 1

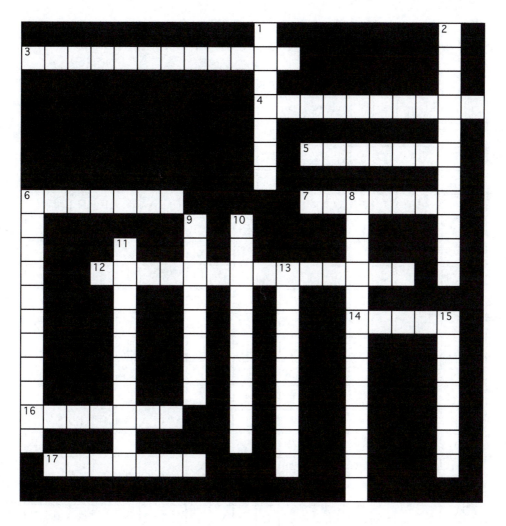

Across

3. Organelles that release energy and are responsible for the chemical reactions that occur in the cell
4. Tiny structures within the cytoplasm of a cell
5. Bone tissue
6. Cell reproduction specific to the ovaries and the testes
7. Another term for internal organs
12. The area in the chest that contains the heart, lungs, and large blood vessels (2 words)
14. Swelling due to fluid in the tissues
16. The study of the structure of the body
17. Complex proteins that increase the speed of a chemical reaction without changing themselves

Down

1. Cell reproduction that results in two daughter cells that are identical to the original cell
2. A state of equilibrium within the body
6. The directional plane that divides the body into left and right halves
8. The ability to permit certain substances to enter and exit through a membrane
9. Same as "one-fourth" of the abdomen
10. The tissue that lines the body cavities and the tubes that lead to the exterior of the body
11. The study of the function of the body
13. Dense connective tissue with elastic qualities
15. Fatty tissue

Name _____

Date _____

Introduction to the Human Body—Puzzle 2

Find the listed words in the puzzle and circle them. (Contains backwards words.)

P	A	V	S	S	N	G	U	G	Q	D	E	M	H	P	D	S	T	M	C
H	U	N	I	F	T	Y	Y	P	C	W	R	L	E	Q	I	M	S	O	O
Y	J	P	A	S	H	K	X	T	N	F	I	X	B	U	I	A	E	R	N
S	A	F	V	T	C	T	X	W	A	C	S	A	N	T	L	L	W	G	N
I	B	W	X	N	O	E	O	L	M	Q	O	D	O	P	B	Z	B	A	E
O	F	M	L	E	O	M	R	B	X	L	T	S	O	A	E	F	P	N	C
L	Y	K	W	Q	K	I	Y	A	C	O	I	T	E	Q	R	C	B	W	T
O	A	J	D	L	V	S	T	A	M	S	Y	M	I	Y	Z	V	K	Y	I
G	O	V	P	L	I	V	D	A	M	C	R	H	V	R	J	N	M	P	V
Y	C	S	T	K	C	G	I	U	R	E	T	C	W	N	D	U	F	J	E
N	E	U	B	E	X	B	S	V	P	D	M	I	I	R	V	L	K	J	Z
M	K	O	K	M	S	C	N	I	Y	B	Y	E	S	C	J	M	W	R	J
J	J	S	M	M	L	S	M	W	R	B	E	H	I	S	G	V	Z	B	W
L	U	M	Z	E	E	E	W	K	U	L	E	Q	E	O	U	T	E	F	C
M	A	Q	J	M	S	J	E	E	C	K	H	I	V	D	S	E	T	S	Y
O	V	S	Y	E	C	U	P	Q	Y	M	T	J	S	Z	E	I	E	B	F
C	F	Z	D	R	M	U	E	H	O	Y	C	V	X	Q	U	V	S	V	M
M	N	E	O	N	I	W	S	H	L	L	J	V	Q	L	K	Q	R	X	Q
E	M	S	X	G	F	L	A	T	L	T	V	V	L	O	N	K	A	E	R
A	E	P	I	T	H	E	L	I	A	L	J	C	S	F	S	L	S	X	N

ANATOMY	MITOSIS
CONNECTIVE	MUSCLE
CYTOPLASM	NERVE
DEHYDRATION	ORGAN
EDEMA	PHYSIOLOGY
ENZYMES	SEMIPERMEABLE
EPITHELIAL	TISSUE
MEIOSIS	VISCERA

Chapter Fourteen
Support, Movement, and Protection: The Skeletal, Muscular, and Integumentary Systems

Objectives

After completing this chapter, you should be able to
do the following:

1. Define and correctly spell each of the key terms.

2. Identify the components of the integumentary system.

3. Name and explain four main functions of the skin.

4. Identify the sections of the skeletal system and describe the function and components of each.

5. Identify and describe three types of joints found within the body.

6. Describe five types of muscle movement.

7. Describe some of the most common diseases that can affect the described systems.

8. Name and describe some of the most common diagnostic tests for diseases of each of the described systems.

Key Terms

- alimentary canal
- appendicular skeleton
- axial skeleton
- constrict
- dilate

- gland
- joint
- peristalsis
- synovial fluid

Chapter Overview

Chapter Fourteen focuses on body systems that have related functions. The skeletal, muscular, and integumentary systems provide support, allow movement, and offer protection. The skeletal system provides the basic framework for the body; the muscles provide shape, support, and movement; and the integumentary system provides shape and protection, and regulates homeostasis.

As a prudent healthcare worker, you must learn the anatomy and physiology of the human body in order to provide competent patient care. Practice saying and writing the terms provided within this chapter. They are words you will need to know to provide proper medical documentation and verbal reports.

Reading Assignment

Read pages 14-1 through 14-18.

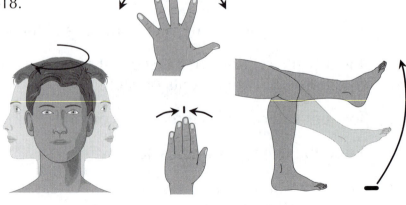

The human body is capable of different types of movement.

Name _____

Date _____

Student Enrichment Activities

Complete the following statements.

1. The two main types of glands contained within the integumentary system are
    _____ and _____.

2. Four functions of the skin are _____, _____,
    _____, and _____.

3. The integumentary system includes _____, _____,
    _____, _____ and _____.

4. _____ _____ is a serious form of skin cancer.

5. The human skeleton contains _____ bones.

6. Bones are made up primarily from two minerals: _____ and
    _____.

7. Name the five functions of the human skeleton.
    A. _____ .
    B. _____ .
    C. _____ .
    D. _____ .
    E. _____ .

8. The skeleton is divided into the _____ and the _____
    sections.

9. Name the four types of bone and provide one example of each:

   A. _____ .

   B. _____ .

   C. _____ .

   D. _____ .

10. Name three kinds of joints and provide one example of each.

    A. _____ .

    B. _____ .

    C. _____ .

11. The body is made up of over _____ muscles.

12. The three kinds of muscle tissue are _____, _____,

    and _____.

13. Name five types of movement of which muscles are capable.

    A. _____   D. _____

    B. _____   E. _____

    C. _____

Unscramble the following terms.

14. SHOASSMEIOT   _____

15. PRATHOY   _____

16. XELIFON   _____

17. SLAMCUE   _____

Name _____

Date _____

18. SUMEHUR   _____

19. SLAPRIESTIS   _____

20. SLUUPTES   _____

21. CAUBSEOSE   _____

22. MEITISLOSTYEO   _____

23. ITALED   _____

24. CNSRTOICT   _____

25. MSYTIISO   _____

Name _____

Date _____

Additional Enrichment Activities

Circle the correct answer.

26. Alopecia, a disease of the integumentary system, is commonly known as:

    A. a bacterial infection.

    B. a fungal infection.

    C. a nail disorder.

    D. baldness.

27. Osteomyelitis is a disorder of the _____ system.

    A. muscular

    B. skeletal

    C. integumentary

    D. none of the above

28. The medical name for a pressure sore is:

    A. a decubitus ulcer.

    B. a burn.

    C. atrophy.

    D. fascia.

29. Another term for striated muscle is:

    A. smooth muscle.

    B. voluntary muscle.

    C. skeletal muscle.

    D. both B and C.

30. The human body contains _____ muscles.

    A. 206

    B. over 600

    C. 500

    D. under 600

31. An example of a type of joint that can be found in the human body is:

    A. a synovial joint.

    B. a fibrous joint.

    C. a cartilaginous joint.

    D. all of the above.

32. The bone in the upper arm is the:

    A. radius.

    B. ulna.

    C. humerus.

    D. femur.

33. Gout is:

    A. a disease of the joints.

    B. a type of fracture.

    C. a debilitating muscular disease.

    D. a soft tissue injury.

34. The wrists and ankles contain examples of _____ joints.

    A. ball and socket

    B. gliding

    C. saddle

    D. hinge

Name _____

Date _____

35. The epidermis has _____ layers.

    A. 3

    B. 1

    C. 5

    D. 6

36. Another name for *sudoriferous* is:

    A. oil.

    B. sweat.

    C. corium.

    D. melanin.

37. The part of the skeletal system made up of the extremities and the shoulder and pelvic girdles is called:

    A. axial.

    B. anterior.

    C. appendicular.

    D. adjointed.

38. *Erythema* is the same as:

    A. fluid overload.

    B. redness of the skin.

    C. a slightly raised rash.

    D. skin vesicles.

39. The group of bones that form the wrist are collectively called:

    A. tarsals.

    B. metacarpals.

    C. metatarsals.

    D. carpals.

Complete the following exercises.

40. List the functions of the skin and explain each one.

_____

_____

_____

_____

_____

_____

_____

_____

_____

_____

41. Describe each main layer of the skin.

_____

_____

_____

_____

_____

_____

Name _____

Date _____

Match the terms in Column A with the appropriate definition in Column B.

Column A

42. _____ epiphysis

43. _____ carpal and tarsal bones

44. _____ malignant melanoma

45. _____ decubitus ulcer

46. _____ dilate

47. _____ striated

48. _____ adduction

49. _____ aspiration

50. _____ red bone marrow

51. _____ fracture

52. _____ maxilla

53. _____ calcaneus

54. _____ muscular system

Column B

A. to enlarge or make bigger

B. provides shape and support for the integumentary system

C. the end of a long bone

D. a crack or break in a bone

E. the heel

F. tissue damage resulting from decreased circulation of blood to a given area

G. short, blocky bones that are closely joined together

H. the soft tissue found in spongy bone that produces all types of blood cells

I. removal or drawing in by suction

J. the movement of a body part toward the middle of the body

K. skeletal or voluntary muscle

L. a fast-spreading skin cancer

M. the upper jaw

Fill in the blanks for each of the following diagrams.

55. Name the bone shapes.

56. The Parts of a Bone

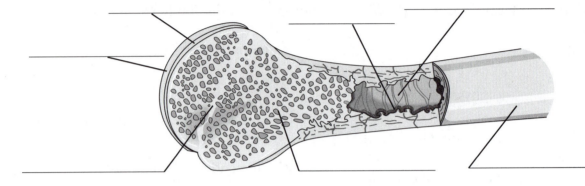

57. The Major Bones of the Skeletal System

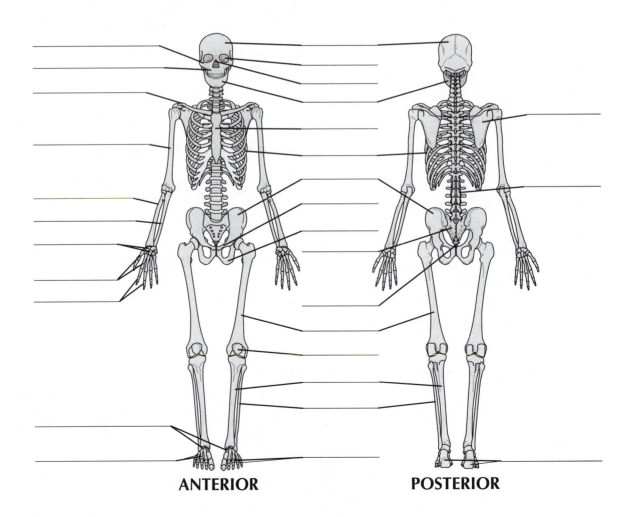

ANTERIOR   **POSTERIOR**

Name _____

Date _____

58. Motion Groups for Joints

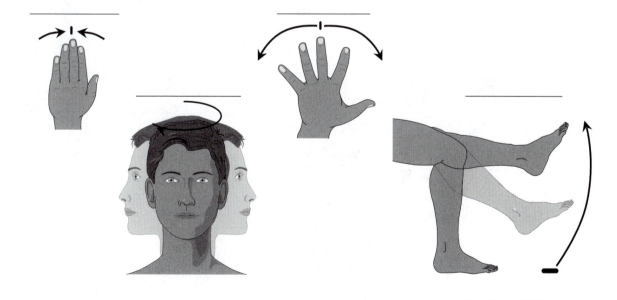

_____   _____   _____

_____   _____   _____

59. Types of Movement

_____   _____

_____   _____

_____

60. The Muscle Types

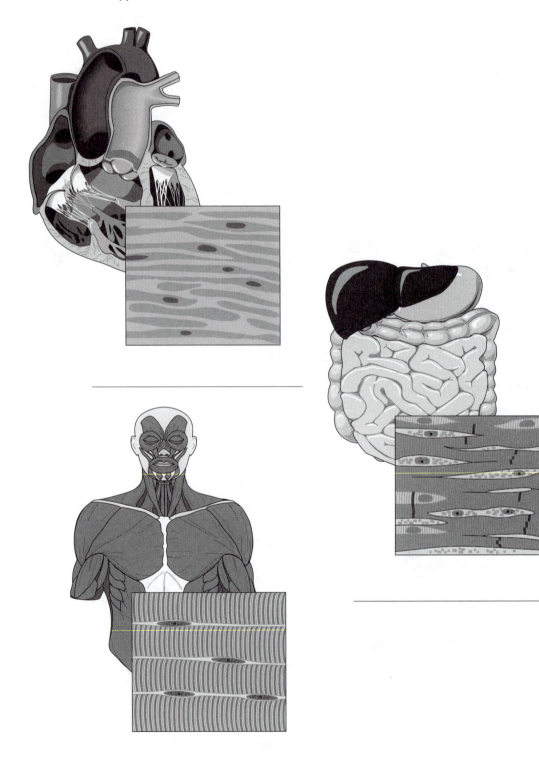

Name _____

Date _____

61.   The Major Muscles of the Body

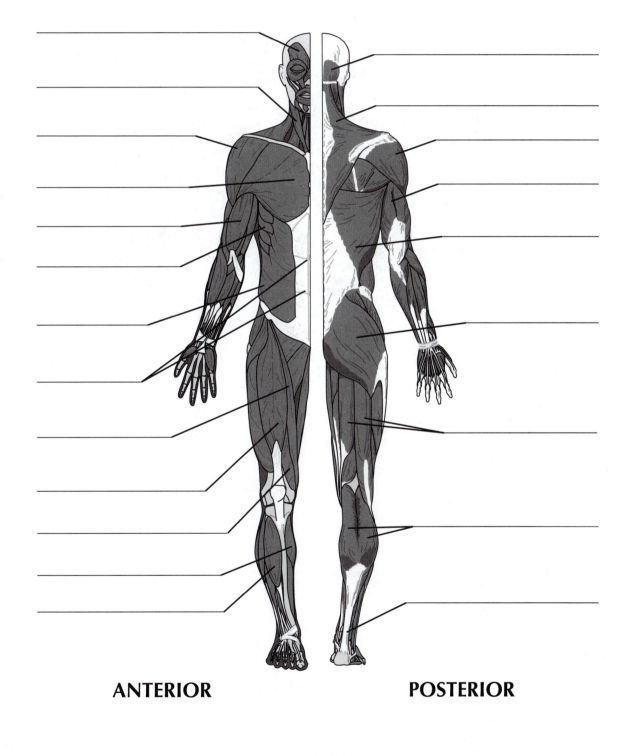

ANTERIOR   **POSTERIOR**

62.   The Parts of the Skin

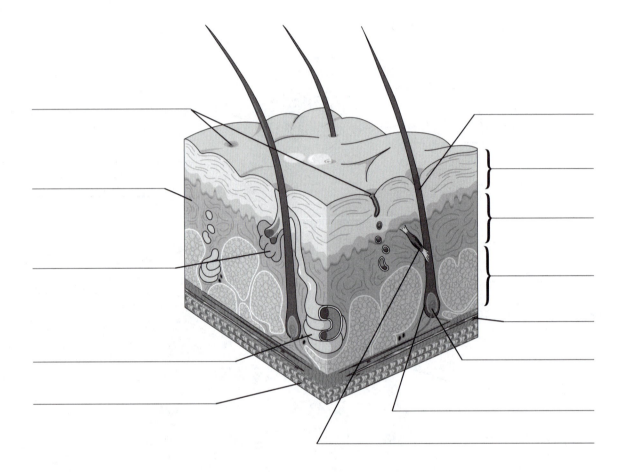

Name _____

Date _____

Support, Movement, and Protection—Puzzle 1

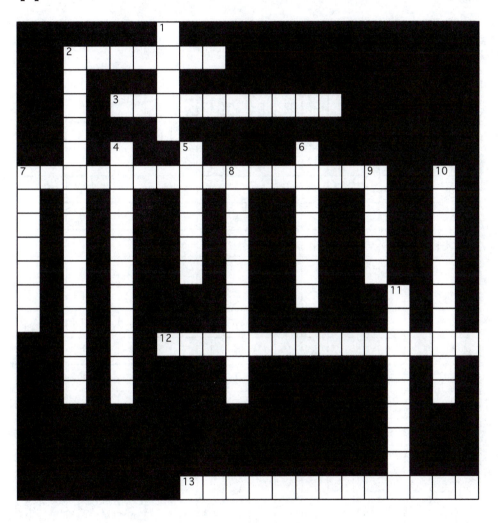

Across

2. The study of the structure of the body
3. The material that fills the medullary canal of bones, and that produces erythrocytes
7. A tissue that supports and attaches other parts to each other (2 words)
12. Fibrous connective tissue located at the distal part of the calf muscle, which secures that muscle to the heel (2 words)
13. Related to the three layers of the skin

Down

1. A place where two or more bones meet
2. A term for the digestive tract (2 words)
4. Rhythmic, wavelike motion that occurs throughout the digestive tract
5. To become larger
6. Bone tissue
7. Pertaining to the heart
8. Tissue that lines the cavities of the body and the principal tubes and passageways that lead to the exterior of the body
9. Swelling due to fluid in the tissues
10. The study of the function of the body
11. To become smaller

Name _____

Date _____

Support, Movement, and Protection—Puzzle 2

Find the listed words in the puzzle and circle them. (Contains backwards words.)

L	A	A	E	T	M	Q	N	X	O	R	N	O	J	A	B	A	R
A	E	D	S	T	F	H	R	F	C	L	L	F	I	M	N	O	A
R	D	T	I	E	A	T	Q	F	Q	D	E	C	U	A	I	W	C
Y	E	V	N	P	L	L	S	K	M	M	S	I	T	R	V	L	N
N	M	I	T	E	O	U	I	A	Z	A	R	O	E	K	V	N	E
X	A	B	H	G	P	S	C	D	F	O	M	T	K	Y	X	S	L
O	U	J	F	W	G	I	E	A	C	Y	N	J	K	J	N	D	B
F	K	F	L	A	M	R	T	S	M	A	C	V	B	J	V	L	I
J	B	S	J	B	B	G	U	H	C	J	Z	L	O	Z	U	W	R
X	W	C	L	M	D	O	C	A	E	A	A	W	M	P	P	Z	W
Y	I	L	Z	W	E	A	L	R	S	L	T	Y	T	N	U	F	L
F	Y	Y	M	S	R	C	V	Y	T	K	I	R	S	R	O	N	D
N	I	J	S	D	A	E	W	H	R	S	Y	A	O	P	G	P	M
W	W	O	I	N	P	U	X	V	D	K	S	Z	L	P	O	H	P
C	B	A	E	A	E	R	S	E	T	Y	N	L	I	E	H	I	X
W	C	U	A	E	F	U	Y	C	O	L	R	Z	D	B	J	Y	B
Y	S	S	Y	S	T	E	M	K	U	D	A	I	R	V	C	A	K
T	P	I	W	D	D	Y	O	N	T	C	I	R	T	S	N	O	C

ACNE	CALCANEUS	EPITHELIAL
ADIPOSE	CARDIAC	FASCIA
ANATOMY	CONSTRICT	LARYNX
ANTERIOR	CORIUM	MACULES
ATROPHY	DILATE	OSSEOUS
BIOPSY	EDEMA	SYSTEM

Chapter Fifteen
Transporting and Transmitting: The Circulatory, Lymphatic, and Nervous Systems

Objectives

After completing this chapter you should be able to
do the following:

1. Define and correctly spell each of the key terms.

2. Name and define the three types of blood vessels and at least four kinds of blood cells.

3. Describe the path of a drop of blood through the body.

4. Identify and explain the diseases that can affect the circulatory, lymphatic, and nervous systems.

5. Describe the common diagnostic tests for the circulatory, lymphatic, and nervous systems.

6. Name the primary functions of the circulatory, lymphatic, and nervous systems.

7. Identify the three nervous systems and their components.

8. List and describe the five main parts of the brain.

Key Terms

- alveoli
- artery
- atrium
- autonomic nervous system
- capillaries
- central nervous system
- cerebrospinal fluid
- gas exchange
- meninges
- motor neurons

- nerve
- parasympathetic nervous system
- peripheral nervous system
- sensory neurons
- sinoatrial node
- somatic nervous system
- sympathetic nervous system
- vein
- ventricle

Chapter Overview

Chapter Fifteen provides a fundamental overview of those systems involved with transporting and transmitting: the circulatory, lymphatic, and nervous systems. Each system is presented in such a way as to encourage learning and memorization.

The circulatory and lymphatic systems are mainly involved with transporting essential substances throughout the body. The nervous system is concerned mainly with transmitting chemical impulses and commands.

Once again, this is a chapter that will require practice using the medical terms in preparation for accurate medical documentation and reporting. For additional assistance, refer to Chapter Twelve in which medical terminology is discussed. Remember, the patient is entitled to receive care from a well-educated and trained healthcare worker.

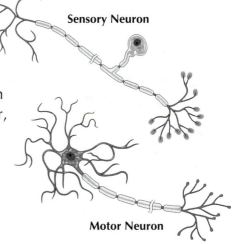

Neurons cause the body to react to its environment.

Reading Assignment

Read pages 15-1 through 15-21.

Name _____

Date _____

Student Enrichment Activities

Complete the following statements.

1. Highly oxygenated blood is transported to the body through _____.

2. The smallest blood vessels in the body are _____.

3. Blood is made up of approximately _____% water.

4. Blood cells that help the blood to clot are called _____.

5. The normal pacemaker of the heart is located in the _____ _____.

6. Name the three layers of cardiac tissue: _____,
   _____, and _____.

7. _____ occurs due to a low oxygen level in the blood in the
   coronary arteries.

8. Impurities are filtered from lymph by the _____ _____.

9. The primary structural units of the nervous system are the _____.

10. _____ neurons are located in the skin and in the sensory organs.

11. _____ neurons originate in the brain and spinal cord and carry
    impulses to the muscles and glands.

12. The brain is surrounded by three layers of membranes called _____.

13. The three layers of meninges are the _____, the _____, and the _____.

14. The _____ nervous system prepares the body for *fight or flight.*

15. The _____ nervous system has a calming effect on the body.

Unscramble the following terms.

16. GREATCLEORADCRIOPHY   _____

17. DOCYMARILA TRAFIONCIN   _____   _____

18. STAMOIC   _____

19. BRIOPTHORMN   _____

20. DRAMIUCRIPE   _____

21. SAIDIENT   _____

22. VIOLEAL   _____

23. SLUVEEN   _____

24. PRESIOUR NEAV AVAC   _____ _____ _____

Name _____

Date _____

25. STINGMIENI _____

26. ANAING _____

27. SPUDIBIC LAVVE _____ _____

28. SCLAUVAR _____

29. PRETENSNYOHI _____

30. MULLEBCREE _____

Name _____

Date _____

Additional Enrichment Activities

Circle the correct answer.

31. Gas exchange means:

    A. oxygen is exchanged for carbon dioxide in the alveoli.

    B. the levels of both gases do not change.

    C. oxygen is exchanged for carbon dioxide in the veins.

    D. none of the above.

32. As a diagnostic term, anemia means:

    A. a low erythrocyte count.

    B. a high leukocyte count.

    C. an accumulation of fat or cholesterol in the arteries.

    D. a high erythrocyte count.

33. There are ____ pairs of cranial nerves.

    A. 31

    B. 33

    C. 4

    D. 12

34. The medulla oblongata is:

    A. part of the central nervous system.

    B. responsible for controlling involuntary functions.

    C. located at the base of the brain.

    D. all of the above.

35. The main cells contained in lymph are:

    A. thrombocytes.

    B. leukocytes.

    C. erythrocytes.

    D. platelets.

36. Alveoli are:

    A. tiny sacs within the lungs where the gas exchange occurs.

    B. tiny tubes within the lungs where the gas exchange occurs.

    C. a blood cell contained only within the lungs.

    D. specialized muscle cells.

37. The peripheral nervous system is subdivided into:

    A. the autonomic nervous system.

    B. the somatic nervous system.

    C. the central nervous system.

    D. both A and B.

38. The parasympathetic nervous system affects the body by:

    A. dilating the pupils.

    B. stimulating gastric juice production.

    C. constricting bronchial tubes.

    D. both B and C.

39. Hemiplegia is:

    A. inflammation of the meninges.

    B. paralysis of one half of the body.

    C. severe pain along the length of a nerve.

    D. disturbed rhythms of the electrical impulses that fire throughout the cerebellum.

Name _____

Date _____

40. Blood is approximately _____ percent water.

    A. 22

    B. 60

    C. 78

    D. 90

41. _____ are the basis of the immune system.

    A. Leukocytes

    B. Plasma

    C. Thrombocytes

    D. Erythrocytes

42. The one-way valve separating the right atrium from the right ventricle is the:

    A. semilunar valve.

    B. pulmonary valve.

    C. mitral valve.

    D. tricuspid valve.

43. The natural pacemaker of the heart is:

    A. the atria.

    B. the sinoatrial node.

    C. the atrium.

    D. the central nervous system.

44. The ventricles of the heart are known as:

    A. receiving chambers.

    B. Purkinji fibers.

    C. pumping chambers.

    D. none of the above.

45. The dura mater is:

   A. the innermost meninge.

   B. the outermost meninge.

   C. a covering of the spinal cord.

   D. both B and C.

46. The spinal cord is an extension of the:

   A. pons.

   B. medulla oblongata.

   C. cerebrum.

   D. cerebellum.

47. The brain has _____ ventricles.

   A. 4

   B. 2

   C. 1

   D. none

48. Angina is a cardiac condition due to:

   A. low levels of carbon dioxide in the blood.

   B. high levels of carbon dioxide in the blood.

   C. hypothermia.

   D. hypoxemia.

49. Phlebitis is:

   A. the inflammation of the inner lining of the heart.

   B. the inflammation of the covering of the brain.

   C. the inflammation of a vein.

   D. the inflammation of a joint.

Name _____

Date _____

50. Muscle coordination and tone, posture, and balance are controlled by:

   A. the cerebellum.

   B. the cerebrum.

   C. the pons.

   D. the midbrain.

51. Chewing and producing saliva are controlled by which area of the brain?

   A. the midbrain

   B. the cerebrum

   C. the cerebellum

   D. the pons

52. Willful actions are controlled by which part of the brain?

   A. the midbrain

   B. the pons

   C. the cerebellum

   D. the cerebrum

53. Sources of lymphatic tissue include:

   A. the bone marrow.

   B. the spleen.

   C. the thymus.

   D. both B and C.

Complete the following exercises.

54. Describe the path of a drop of blood through the body, beginning with the superior vena cava.

_____

_____

_____

_____

_____

_____

_____

55. Define each of the following terms.

    A. erythrocytes: _____

    _____

    B. hemoglobin: _____

    _____

    C. thrombocytes: _____

    _____

    D. leukocytes: _____

    _____

    E. artery: _____

    _____

    F. capillaries: _____

    _____

    G. vein: _____

    _____

    H. gas exchange: _____

    _____

    I. antibodies: _____

    _____

Name _____

Date _____

56. Describe the anatomy of the heart.

_____

_____

_____

_____

_____

_____

57. Describe four conditions that affect the lymphatic system.

_____

_____

_____

_____

_____

58. Describe sensory and motor neurons.

_____

_____

_____

_____

_____

59. Describe each of the following.

A. central nervous system: _____

_____

_____

B. peripheral nervous system: _____

_____

_____

60. Describe the effects of the two divisions of the autonomic nervous system on each of the organs listed.

Parasympathetic Nervous System	Sympathetic Nervous System

A. bladder: _____

B. heart: _____

C. lungs: _____

D. pupils: _____

61. Define the following terms.

A. hemiplegia: _____

_____

B. concussion: _____

_____

C. CVA: _____

_____

D. epilepsy: _____

_____

_____

E. neuralgia: _____

_____

Name _____

Date _____

Fill in the blanks for each of the following diagrams.

62. Types of Blood Cells

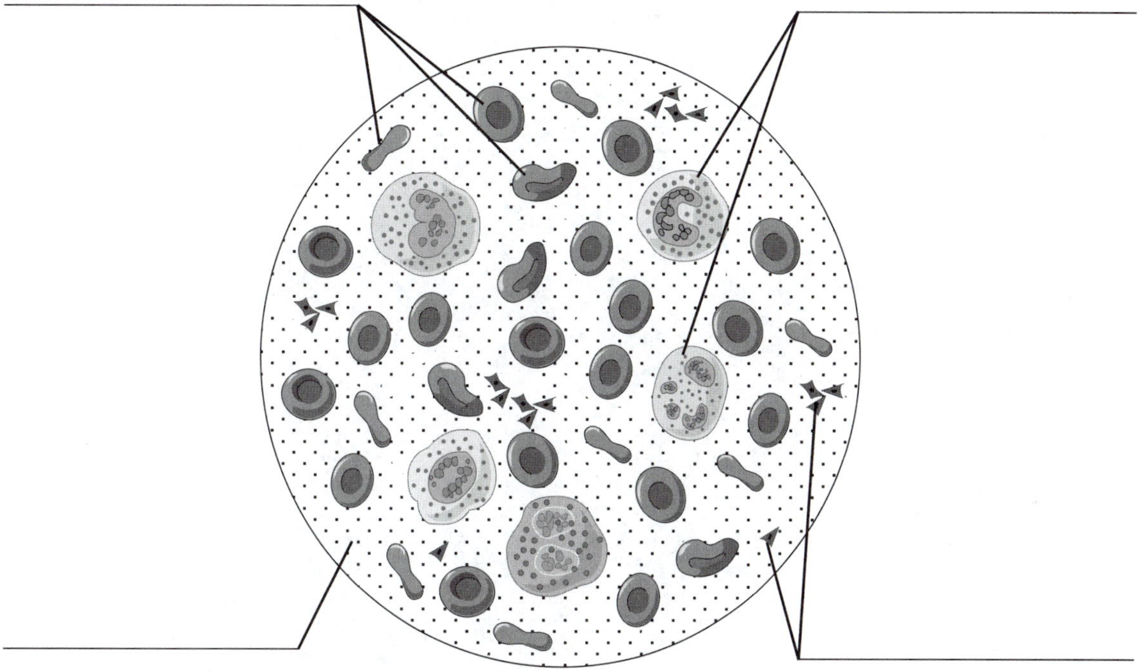

63. The Anterior Heart

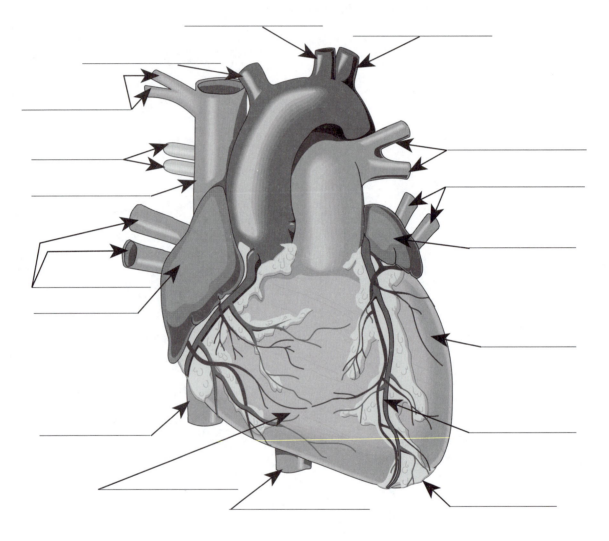

Name _____

Date _____

64. The Circulatory Path

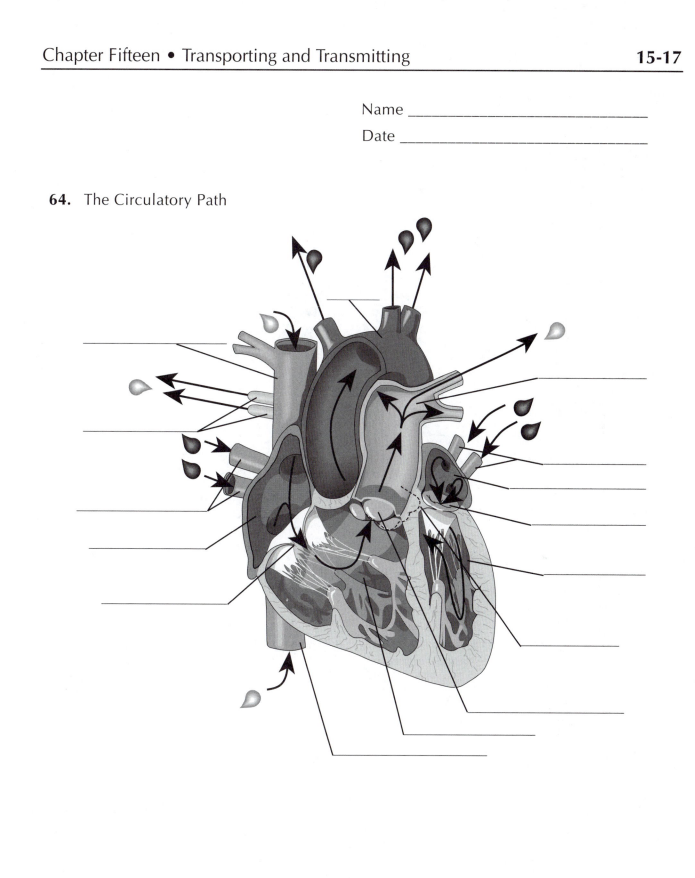

65. The Lymphatic System

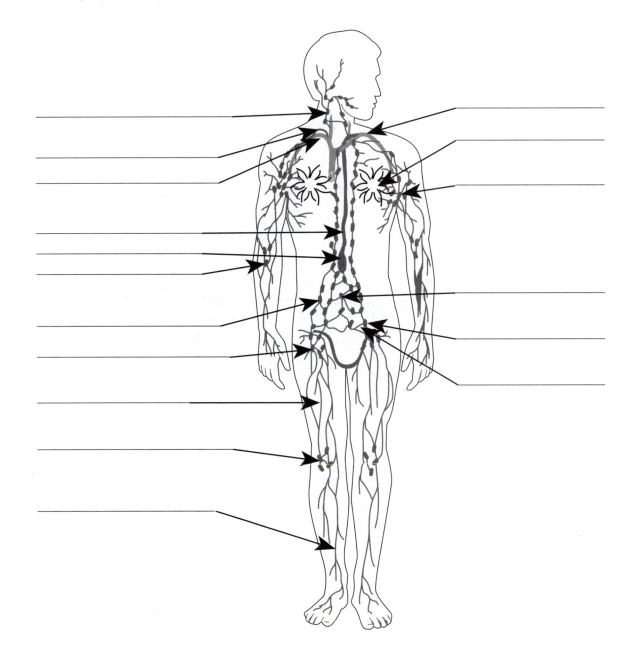

Name _____

Date _____

66. Neurons

SENSORY NEURON

MOTOR NEURON

67. Lateral View of the Brain

68. The Autonomic Nervous System

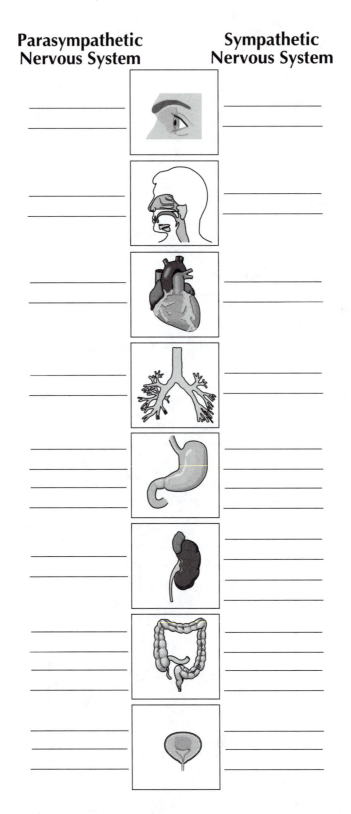

Parasympathetic Nervous System   **Sympathetic Nervous System**

Name _____

Date _____

Transporting and Transmitting—Puzzle 1

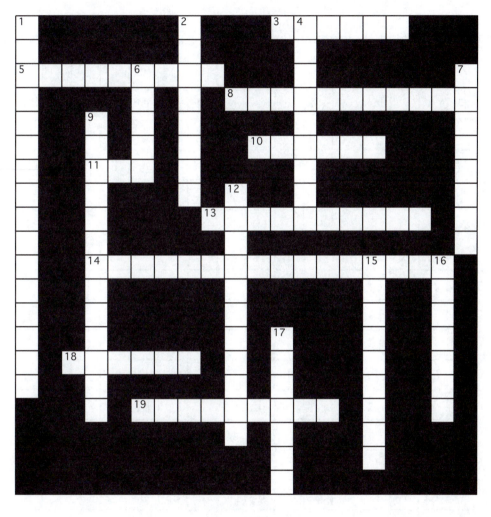

Across

3. A reduction in red blood cells or the amount of hemoglobin in the blood
5. The outer layer of the meninges
8. The one-way valve located between the left atrium and left ventricle of the heart (2 words)
10. The organ in the upper left quadrant that produces lymphocytes and monocytes
11. The abbreviation for cerebrovascular accident
13. The thick, muscular layer of the heart
14. The principle vein that drains deoxygenated blood from the lower body into the right atrium (3 words)
18. The fluid portion of the blood
19. Relating to the lungs

Down

1. The lower portion of the brain stem that controls involuntary actions (2 words)
2. Inflammation of the lymph nodes
4. Severe pain along the length of a nerve
6. The main artery in the body
7. The area of the brain that controls willfull actions
9. Another name for the mitral valve (2 words)
12. An abnormally low blood pressure
15. A soft tissue injury caused by seepage of blood into tissue
16. Microscopic air sacs in the lungs where the exchange of oxygen and carbon dioxide occurs
17. Pertaining to the body

Name _____

Date _____

Transporting and Transmitting—Puzzle 2

Find the listed words in the puzzle and circle them. (Contains backwards words.)

C	S	C	A	R	T	E	R	I	O	L	E	S	A	N	A
P	I	E	A	Z	Q	I	V	X	P	D	U	C	A	L	T
E	T	M	T	R	C	A	Y	B	C	I	L	N	V	U	P
R	M	B	E	Y	D	C	F	D	O	B	I	E	N	B	L
I	U	Y	A	T	C	I	K	Z	G	G	O	I	Y	B	A
C	I	H	T	M	S	O	O	B	N	L	C	Z	Y	S	T
A	D	R	S	Y	E	Y	R	A	I	A	X	B	R	P	E
R	R	B	Q	A	F	V	S	H	I	O	W	C	B	X	L
D	A	Z	D	T	I	T	S	N	T	R	K	W	N	C	E
I	C	I	D	P	H	I	T	E	V	Y	V	J	C	W	T
U	O	N	L	Y	T	I	Y	D	C	E	R	N	I	M	S
M	Y	A	M	I	M	N	I	Q	F	Q	N	E	O	Y	H
D	M	U	N	A	O	B	Q	V	E	W	P	U	T	X	N
P	S	E	L	Q	P	O	U	S	C	O	C	B	L	H	A
F	D	L	E	U	K	O	C	Y	T	E	S	O	U	E	R
A	A	O	R	T	I	C	V	A	L	V	E	L	F	U	S

ADENITIS	LEUKOCYTES
ALVEOLI	MYOCARDIUM
ANGINA	PERICARDIUM
AORTIC VALVE	PLATELETS
ARTERIOLES	SYSTEMIC
AXON	THYMUS
CARDIO	TUNICA INTIMA
ERYTHROCYTES	VENULES

Chapter Sixteen
Excretion: The Respiratory, Digestive, and Urinary Systems

Objectives

After completing this chapter you should be able to
do the following:

1. Define and correctly spell each of the key terms.

2. Identify and describe all the parts of the respiratory system.

3. Describe the breathing process.

4. Describe at least four diagnostic tests for the respiratory system.

5. Name two enzymes produced in the stomach.

6. Trace the course of a bite of food through the entire digestive system.

7. Name and explain at least three functions of the liver.

8. Name the three enzymes produced by the pancreas.

9. Briefly explain the disease process of diabetes.

10. Describe the three main functions of the kidneys.

11. Describe the path of a drop of urine as it passes through the urinary system.

Key Terms

- alveoli
- chyme
- cilia
- diaphragm
- insulin
- kidneys
- larynx
- metabolism
- nephron

- pancreas
- peristalsis
- trachea
- ulcer
- ureter
- urinary bladder
- ventilation
- vermiform appendix
- vocal folds

Chapter Overview

You are now beginning the study of the systems involved with excretion: the respiratory, digestive, and urinary systems. Every system in the human body is intricately dependent upon every other system. As you will recall, the anatomy and physiology of the body must be in harmony with each other in order to maintain homeostasis.

At the conclusion of this chapter, you will have studied the fundamental anatomy and physiology of nine body systems. It is vitally important that you continue to review each system and begin to recognize how the human body functions *as a whole.*

Reading Assignment

Read pages 16-1 through 16-21.

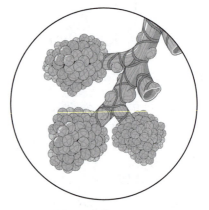

Carbon dioxide (CO_2) and oxygen (O_2) easily pass through the capillary walls that surround the alveoli. It is within these structures that gas exchange occurs.

Name _____

Date _____

Student Enrichment Activities

Complete the following statements.

1. The body stores enough oxygen for _____ minutes.

2. Name the parts of the respiratory system: _____,

    _____, _____, _____,

    _____, _____, and the _____.

3. The voice box, or _____, is made up of _____ layers of cartilage.

4. The largest organs of the respiratory system are the _____.

5. The thoracic cavity is separated from the abdominal cavity by the _____.

6. The term _____ means respiration.

7. The respiratory center is located in the _____ _____.

8. A lung disease characterized by wheezing is known as _____.

9. _____ is the enzyme contained in saliva.

10. The stomach is capable of holding a _____ _____ of food and liquid.

11. The main components of the digestive secretions in the stomach are

    _____ _____ and _____.

12. Food generally remains in the stomach for _____ minutes to _____ hours.

13. The small intestine is about _____ _____ long when uncoiled.

14. The large intestine is approximately _____ _____ long.

15. The vermiform appendix is attached to the _____.

16. List four functions of the large intestine:

    A. _____

    B. _____

    C. _____

    D. _____

17. Four functions of the liver are:

    _____

    _____ .

18. Produced by the pancreas, _____ is released into the bloodstream according to the amount of circulating glucose.

19. A _____ is a needle puncture of the abdominal cavity followed by aspiration of fluid.

20. The primary component of urine is _____.

21. The kidneys produce about _____ of urine daily.

22. List the three main functions of the kidneys:

    A. _____

    B. _____

    C. _____

Name _____

Date _____

23. The urge to urinate occurs when the bladder contains approximately _____ _____ of urine.

Unscramble the following terms.

24. SHRIOCRIS   _____

25. TENCICONNIEN   _____

26. SLAMYEA   _____

27. LANAS STUMEP   _____   _____

28. SLAISPREITS   _____

29. VENATRSERS LONCO   _____   _____

30. MIGDIOS LONCO   _____   _____

31. SLATECAL   _____

32. SPRANCEA   _____

33. SPAILE   _____

34. TIEXISASP   _____

35. NYDSEAP   _____

Name _____

Date _____

Additional Enrichment Activities

Circle the correct answer.

36. The scientific name for the Adam's Apple is the:

    A. vocal cords.

    B. vocal folds.

    C. cricothyroid cartilage.

    D. thyroid cartilage.

37. Food traveling through the alimentary canal takes as long as:

    A. 36 hrs.

    B. 4 to 20 hrs.

    C. 30 min to 4 hrs.

    D. 5 to 7 days.

38. Water can be stored by the human body for:

    A. 4 to 6 hrs.

    B. 36 hrs.

    C. weeks.

    D. 5 to 7 days.

39. The scientific name for the voice box is the:

    A. trachea.

    B. vocal folds.

    C. larynx.

    D. vocal cords.

40. The main muscle that adults use for breathing is the:

    A. intercostal.

    B. diaphragm.

    C. abdominal.

    D. trapezius.

41. Cellular respiration is:

    A. internal respiration.

    B. external respiration.

    C. the first phase of ventilation.

    D. the respiratory cycle.

42. The _____ is located in the left upper quadrant.

    A. left lobe of the liver

    B. gall bladder

    C. pancreas

    D. both A and C

43. Healthy kidneys produce approximately _____ of urine per day.

    A. 1500 cc to 2000 cc

    B. 1 $\frac{1}{2}$ to 2 gallons

    C. 1 $\frac{1}{2}$ to 2 quarts

    D. both A and C

44. Waste products are filtered from the blood in the:

    A. neuron.

    B. nephrons.

    C. spleen.

    D. gallbladder.

Name _____

Date _____

45. The three enzymes produced in the stomach are:

    A. pepsin, renin, bile.

    B. lipase, lactase, sucrase.

    C. pepsin, bile, amylopsin.

    D. pepsin, lipase, rennin.

46. Lactase, maltase, and sucrase are:

    A. liver enzymes.

    B. intestinal enzymes.

    C. stomach enzymes.

    D. pancreatic enzymes.

47. The hormone produced by the islets of Langerhans is called:

    A. insulin.

    B. bile.

    C. ptyalin.

    D. epinephrine.

48. Pancreatic juice and bile are secreted into the:

    A. jejunum.

    B. stomach.

    C. large intestine.

    D. duodenum.

49. The right lung has ____ lobes.

    A. 2

    B. 6

    C. 3

    D. 5

50. The thin layer of tissue surrounding each lung is the:

    A. periosteum.

    B. pleura.

    C. perineum.

    D. pericardium.

51. The epiglottis is located:

    A. superior to the glottis.

    B. lateral to the glottis.

    C. medial to the glottis.

    D. inferior to the glottis.

52. Bile is helpful in:

    A. producing heparin.

    B. producing erythrocytes.

    C. breaking down fats.

    D. being a waste product, bile has no significant function.

53. The urge to urinate is normally perceived when _____ of urine is in the bladder.

    A. 1 cup

    B. 250 cc

    C. 500 cc

    D. 16 ounces

54. Peristalsis occurs in the:

    A. ureters.

    B. esophagus.

    C. intestines.

    D. all of the above.

Name _____

Date _____

55. Inflammation of the kidneys is called:

  A. nephritis.

  B. pyelonephritis.

  C. neuritis.

  D. cystitis.

Complete the following exercises.

56. Describe five functions of the liver.

  _____

  _____

  _____

  _____

  _____

  _____

57. Explain the location and functions of cilia.

  _____

  _____

  _____

  _____

  _____

58. Describe a bronchoscopy.

  _____

  _____

  _____

  _____

  _____

Match the terms in Column A with the appropriate definition in Column B.

Column A

59. _____ ventilation

60. _____ pleura

61. _____ chyme

62. _____ ulcer

63. _____ ptyalin

64. _____ pleurisy

65. _____ nephrons

66. _____ IVP

67. _____ hematuria

68. _____ polyuria

69. _____ atelectasis

70. _____ pulmonary function tests

Column B

A. inflammation of the pleura

B. the functional units of the kidney

C. the exchange of air between the lungs and the atmosphere

D. excessive urination

E. the presence of blood in urine

F. a lesion on the skin or mucous membrane accompanied by sloughing of inflamed, dead skin

G. abbreviation for intravenous pyelogram

H. tests used to determine the capacity of the lungs to take in O_2 and release CO_2

I. the thin layer of tissue that surrounds each lung and extends over the diaphragm and walls of the thorax

J. an enzyme found in saliva that breaks down starches into simple sugars

K. a semisolid mass found in the stomach formed by the mixture of gastric secretions and food

L. airless lung tissue; collapsed lung

Name _____

Date _____

71. Define each of the following terms.

A. endoscopy: _____

_____

B. upper GI series: _____

_____

C. paracentesis: _____

_____

72. Describe the journey of a piece of food through the alimentary canal.

_____

_____

_____

_____

_____

_____

_____

_____

73. Describe the process of breathing.

_____

_____

_____

_____

_____

_____

_____

_____

Fill in the blanks for each of the following diagrams.

74. The Respiratory Tract

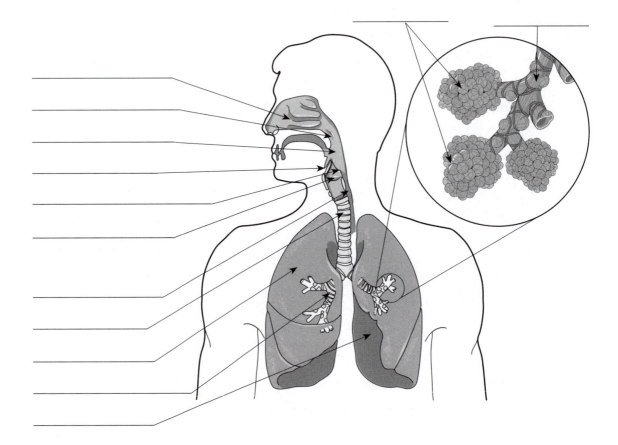

Name _____

Date _____

75. Cellular Respiration

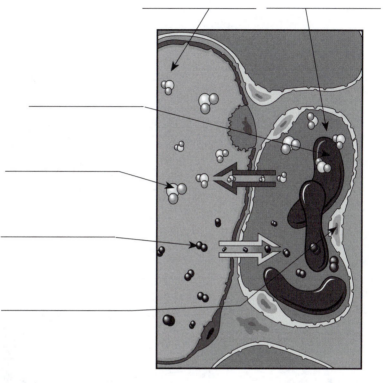

76. Digestive Juices and their Enzymes.

Digestive Juices and Their Enzymes				
Juice	**Gland**	**Place of Action**	**Enzymes**	**Effect on Foods**
Saliva				
Gastric Juice				
Pancreatic Juice				
Intestinal Juice				
Bile				

77.   The Digestive System

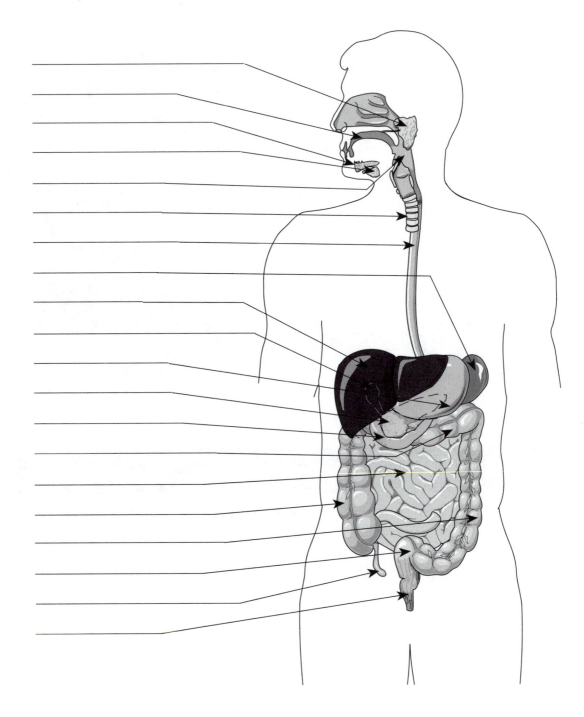

Name _____

Date _____

78. The Urinary System (Male)

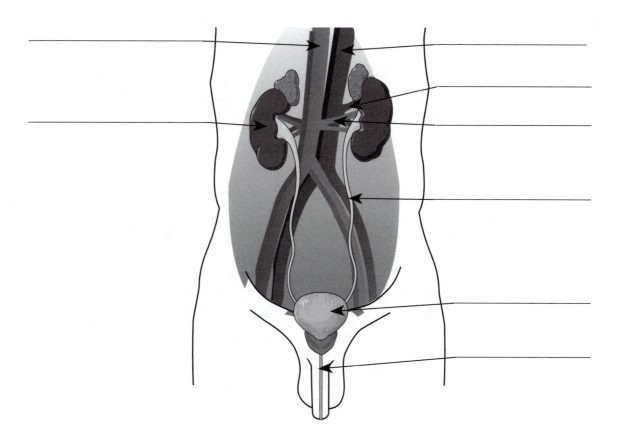

79. A Simplified Nephron

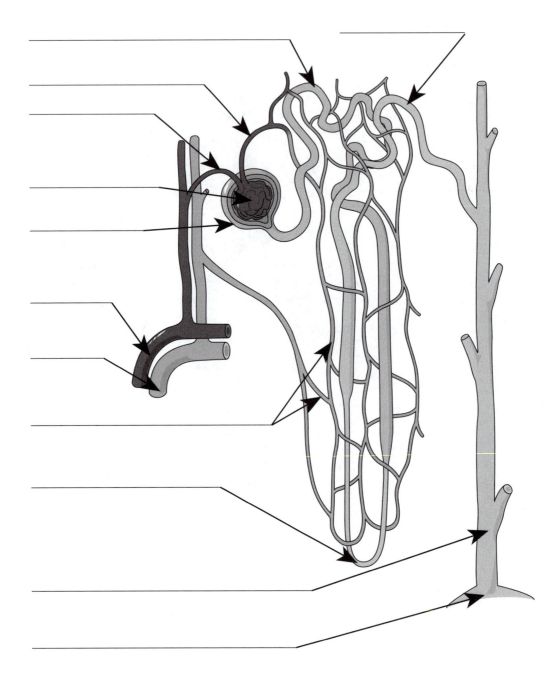

Name _____

Date _____

Excretion—Puzzle 1

Across

3. A lack of oxygen
7. The throat
8. Difficult or painful breathing, shortness of breath
10. The tube that transports urine from the bladder
13. A corpuscle at the end of a nephron that contains the glomerulus (2 words)
18. Upper respiratory infection
19. The windpipe, a tube of cartilage extending from the larynx to the bronchial tubes
23. Inflammation of the lining of the nasal cavity
24. The presence of blood in urine

Down

1. Inflammation of the lungs
2. The organ that produces insulin and aids in digestion
4. The voice box
5. An enzyme that helps break down fats
6. A highly communicable disease of the upper respiratory tract
9. Smaller portions of the bronchi
11. Inflammation of the liver
12. The last section of the small intestine
14. Inflammation of the urinary bladder
15. A chronic lung disease that destroys the alveoli
16. Finger-like projections found on membrane surfaces
17. Stones usually made up of mineral salts
20. Microscopic air sacs in the lungs
21. The outer layer of an organ such as the kidney
22. Causes breathing difficulty, wheezing, and coughing

Name _____

Date _____

Excretion—Puzzle 2

Find the listed words in the puzzle and circle them. (Contains backwards words.)

D	M	L	V	F	D	Q	V	D	G	U	B	T	E	E	F
I	X	U	I	I	J	P	S	N	D	D	Y	N	S	I	T
A	Q	B	N	P	L	C	T	G	T	I	I	A	B	Y	O
L	P	S	R	U	A	L	Q	H	Y	P	L	R	V	I	Y
Y	J	V	Q	O	J	S	I	L	U	Y	I	A	L	P	I
S	B	Y	N	J	N	E	E	S	M	N	I	E	C	J	W
I	H	T	I	P	N	C	J	A	O	O	Z	T	S	T	S
S	W	F	E	A	I	Z	H	G	C	M	Z	X	B	G	I
M	Q	X	V	I	R	N	E	I	A	E	V	C	E	I	T
C	Q	I	Q	A	O	N	L	M	O	R	C	B	U	X	I
A	L	C	I	R	A	W	A	W	O	L	H	U	D	M	N
P	F	L	H	I	T	Z	C	V	W	C	E	T	M	V	I
Y	I	P	X	K	L	H	Z	W	N	R	W	S	E	M	H
C	E	O	Y	L	Q	L	J	D	J	R	F	U	N	R	R
N	N	H	E	M	A	T	U	R	I	A	Z	T	G	Q	U
A	E	N	D	O	S	C	O	P	Y	Z	Z	T	P	W	G

AMYLASE	HEMATURIA
ANOXIA	JEJUNUM
BRONCHIOLES	LIPASE
CECUM	NEPHRON
CILIA	RHINITIS
DIALYSIS	SUPINE
ENDOSCOPY	URETHRA
FIBRINOGEN	VILLI

Chapter Seventeen
The Specialties: The Sensory, Endocrine, and Reproductive Systems

Objectives

After completing this chapter you should be able to
do the following:

1. Define and correctly spell each of the key terms.

2. Identify the five major senses.

3. Explain how sound waves are transmitted, received, and interpreted.

4. Explain how the process of smelling occurs.

5. Identify the four kinds of taste receptors.

6. Name the two types of glands and their secretions.

7. Identify the glands within the endocrine system.

8. Explain the function of insulin.

9. Explain the function of estrogen.

10. Explain the function of testosterone.

11. Name the parts of the female and male reproductive systems.

12. Name four sexually transmitted diseases.

Key Terms

- auditory nerve
- circumcision
- endocrine
- estrogen
- exocrine
- gland
- menstruation

- sexually transmitted diseases
- taste receptors
- testes
- testosterone
- uterus
- vulva

Chapter Overview

In order for the body to perform at its optimal level, each part of every system must be in a complete state of wellness. Chapter Seventeen introduces three special systems of the body: the sensory, endocrine, and reproductive systems.

This chapter completes the overview of basic anatomy and physiology you will need as you begin your career in healthcare. Remember, frequent review of the other systems will help you understand how the parts of the body work together as a unit.

The patient deserves a healthcare worker who understands the human body. Such knowledge is fundamental to your ability to assist in treatment methods as well as plans of care.

Reading Assignment

Read pages 17-1 through 17-23.

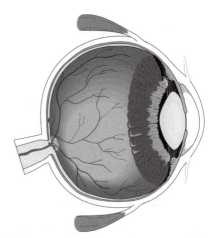

Sight is one of the major senses. The others are hearing, taste, smell, and touch.

Name _____

Date _____

Student Enrichment Activities

Complete the following statements.

1. Name the three layers of the eyeball: the _____, the
    _____ _____, and the _____.

2. There are approximately _____ extraocular muscles that coordinate eye movement.

3. The two types of nerve cells contained within the retina are called
    _____ and _____.

4. The ear is responsible for _____ and _____.

5. The three ossicles are the _____, _____, and
    the _____.

6. List the ten endocrine glands.

    _____

    _____

7. A chronic disease characterized by elongation and enlargement of the bones is
    _____.

8. The body's metabolism is regulated by the _____ gland and the
    hormones secreted by the pituitary gland.

9. _____ is a hormone produced by the pancreas.

10. The sex glands of the female are the _____.

11. The primary hormone produced by the ovaries is _____.

12. The pear-shaped muscular organ located within the female abdominal cavity is the _____.

13. Name the parts of the male reproductive system: (Hint: There are nine.)

    _____

    _____

14. The mixture of sperm and other fluid substances is called_____.

Unscramble the following terms.

15. SCRIOMCIUCIN   _____

16. UHCGSINS ISEDSAE   _____ _____

17. STROETOSTENE   _____

18. SNILUIN   _____

19. OOOETSPC   _____

20. CLEANPAT   _____

21. SLIMENA CLEVESIS   _____ _____

22. MENIREPU   _____

Name _____

Date _____

23. LCTTNAAIO   _____

24. SAV SNERFEDE   _____   _____

25. GROESTEN   _____

26. REACON   _____

27. REMUCEN   _____

28. ATRIUMDOEY   _____

29. PECOTIC GRANPENCY   _____   _____

30. CHLEACO   _____

Name _____

Date _____

Additional Enrichment Activities

Circle the correct answer.

31. The master gland of the human body is the:

   A. thyroid gland.

   B. pituitary gland.

   C. adrenal gland.

   D. sex glands.

32. In order for the thyroid gland to produce hormones, it requires:

   A. potassium.

   B. sodium.

   C. magnesium.

   D. iodine.

33. Cones are nerve receptors found in the:

   A. retina.

   B. inner ear.

   C. middle ear.

   D. cornea.

34. Rods are used for:

   A. dark or dim light.

   B. bright light.

   C. production of ptyalin.

   D. equilibrium.

35. The spherical shape of the eyeball is due to the:
    A. aqueous humor.
    B. rods and cones.
    C. vitreous humor.
    D. six muscle groups.

36. Cataracts affect the:
    A. conjunctiva.
    B. stapes, incus, and malleus.
    C. tympanic membrane.
    D. lens.

37. The _____ _____ transmits sound waves to the brain for interpretation:
    A. eustachian tube.
    B. auditory nerve.
    C. tympanic membrane.
    D. semicircular canals.

38. A *popping* sensation in the ear results from:
    A. sinusitis.
    B. rhinitis.
    C. vestibular nerve dysfunction.
    D. unequal pressure between the outer and inner ear.

39. The gland located on the anterior trachea is the:
    A. parathyroid.
    B. thymus.
    C. thyroid.
    D. pineal body.

Name _____

Date _____

40. An example of an exocrine gland is:

   A. a sebaceous gland.

   B. an ovary.

   C. the pancreas.

   D. an adrenal gland.

41. The primary hormone secreted by the ovaries is:

   A. progesterone.

   B. thyroid.

   C. estrogen.

   D. depo provera.

42. Collectively, the external genitalia of females is called:

   A. the vulva.

   B. the uvula.

   C. the perineum.

   D. all of the above.

Complete the following exercises.

43. Describe two main functions of the uterus.

   _____

   _____

   _____

44. List the anatomical parts of the female reproductive system.

_____

_____

_____

_____

45. Describe Cushing's disease and Addison's disease.

_____

_____

_____

_____

_____

_____

_____

46. Describe the process of hearing a sound.

_____

_____

_____

_____

_____

_____

_____

47. List the five major senses.

_____

_____

_____

Name _____

Date _____

48. Identify and describe the three protective tissue layers of the eye.

_____

_____

_____

_____

_____

49. Explain why the ear and the throat are susceptible to infections.

_____

_____

_____

_____

50. Define the following terms.

A. glaucoma: _____

_____

B. cataract: _____

_____

C. astigmatism: _____

_____

D. otitis media: _____

_____

E. goiter: _____

_____

F. hyperthyroidism: _____

_____

G. diabetes mellitus: _____

_____

_____

H. sexually transmitted disease: _____

_____

Fill in the blanks for each of the following diagrams.

51. The Eye

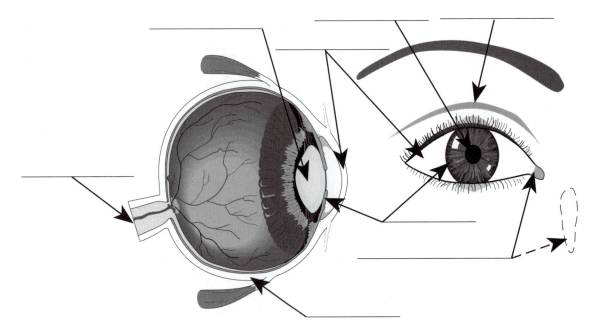

Name _____

Date _____

52. The Ear

53. How Sound is Heard

54. The Taste Receptors

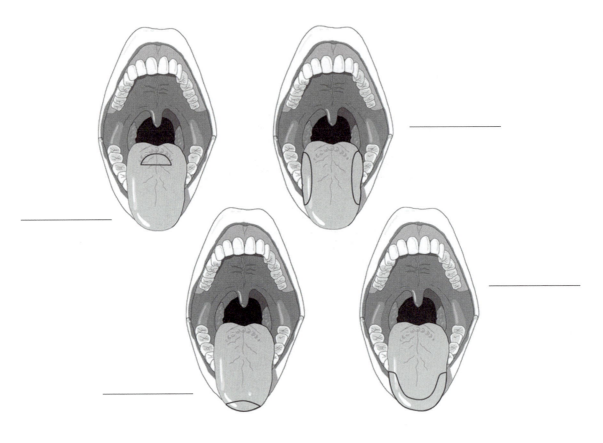

Name _____

Date _____

55. The Endocrine System

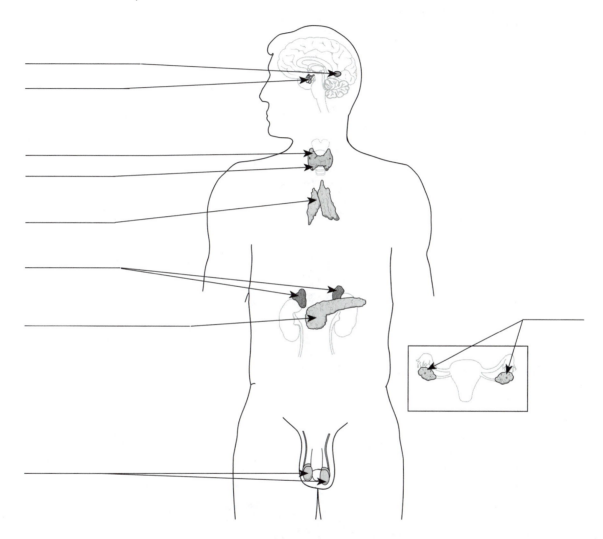

56. The Female Reproductive System (Anterior View)

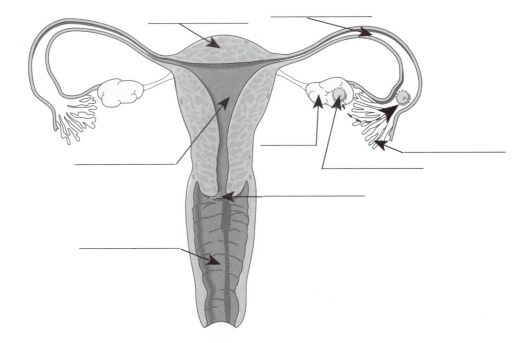

57. The Female Reproductive System (Lateral View)

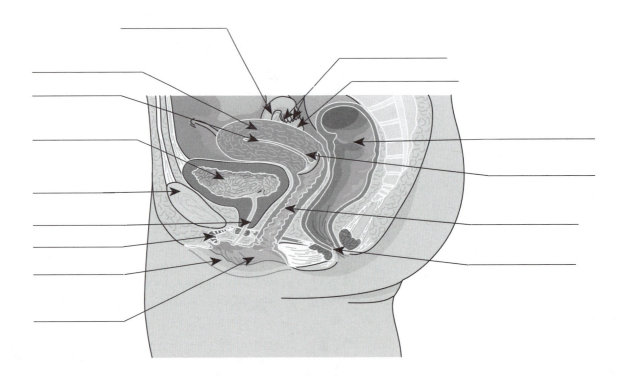

Name _____

Date _____

58. The Male Reproductive System (Lateral View)

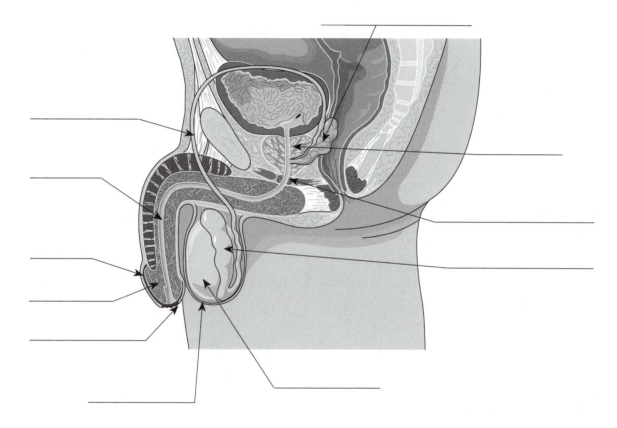

Name _____

Date _____

The Specialties—Puzzle 1

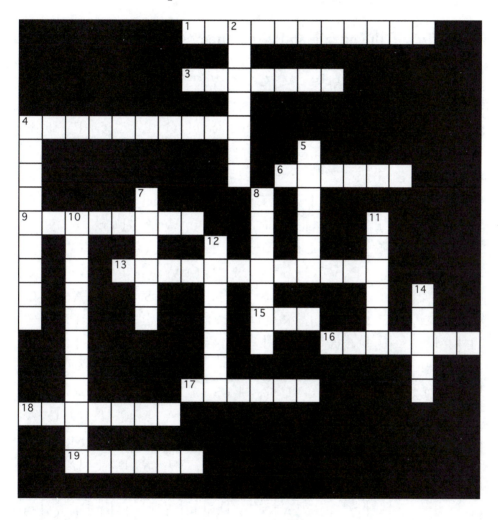

Across

1. The two lips of adipose tissue on either side of the vaginal opening (2 words)
3. The foreskin of the penis
4. The coiled tube next to the testes that stores sperm until they are mature and active
6. The neck of the uterus that protrudes into the vagina
9. The loss of transparency of the lens of the eye
13. The surgical removal of the foreskin of the penis
15. Abbreviation for sexually transmitted disease
16. A hormone secreted by the pancreas that causes glucose to leave the bloodstream and enter the cell
17. The innermost membrane of the eye
18. The female sex glands
19. To become larger

Down

2. The mammary glands that produce milk after the birth of a child
4. Pertaining to a gland that secretes hormones directly into the bloodstream
5. A viral infection, can be a sexually transmitted disease
7. A muscular tube in females that forms the passageway between the cervix and the vulva
8. A simple sugar used to produce energy
10. A structure in the chest that produces lymphocytes and antibodies in early life (2 words)
11. The main part or base of a hollow organ
12. The outer or external portion of the ear
14. The female external genitalia

Name _____

Date _____

The Specialties—Puzzle 2

Find the listed words in the puzzle and circle them. (Contains backwards words.)

M	Y	Y	D	X	B	G	E	M	C	Q	W	T	J	E	H	H	C	P	S
Z	Y	E	V	B	C	J	C	R	X	C	A	K	L	N	R	U	T	I	C
X	H	O	C	E	S	B	T	K	A	C	R	U	G	E	G	O	P	N	L
N	I	I	P	K	B	N	G	L	T	N	B	E	J	U	V	H	J	N	E
H	V	V	E	I	S	Z	A	I	E	I	N	E	I	R	X	E	L	A	R
V	G	S	R	X	A	S	L	M	T	I	U	C	W	U	V	X	T	X	A
E	O	A	U	E	E	E	U	S	R	D	Q	C	W	A	J	H	T	N	A
E	V	R	C	P	C	R	E	C	W	I	E	K	M	I	M	S	O	M	C
U	B	V	R	R	E	V	O	B	Y	M	P	O	W	N	I	Z	W	X	Z
T	V	E	K	C	O	D	B	R	N	Y	N	B	V	S	Q	F	A	C	O
A	H	U	E	E	N	M	L	R	D	L	X	X	R	E	H	C	T	N	Z
E	R	A	S	E	N	W	E	A	E	A	S	I	G	H	F	K	I	D	N
J	D	R	Q	T	Q	K	T	G	C	A	F	F	Q	Q	W	D	M	R	P
A	I	L	W	U	J	J	G	C	A	T	S	E	K	O	K	P	R	U	R
K	S	C	E	H	H	S	W	S	Y	L	A	T	A	B	Q	P	O	D	A
O	P	J	V	N	M	X	P	X	J	R	Y	T	S	R	Z	B	M	O	Y
E	J	E	T	J	U	X	K	K	W	R	I	A	I	R	B	J	U	C	J
F	P	V	N	W	W	O	B	R	E	I	I	S	T	O	H	M	T	Q	V
V	N	I	L	M	D	W	W	A	K	Z	V	B	B	T	N	F	I	O	O
S	E	M	E	N	H	Q	K	T	N	S	M	V	O	H	G	L	U	F	P

ACROMEGALY
BREASTS
CERUMEN
CERVIX
ENDOCRINE
FIMBRAE
HERPES
LACTATION

MYOPIA
PINNA
SCLERA
SEMEN
TACTILE
TUMOR
VESTIBULE

Chapter Eighteen
Basic First Aid

Objectives

After completing this chapter you should be able to
do the following:

1. Define and correctly spell each of the key terms.

2. Describe how to perform the primary survey.

3. Identify the two ways to open an airway.

4. Describe the two ways to control hemorrhage from a
    traumatic injury.

5. Describe the basic procedure for performing a secondary survey.

6. List at least three signs that a person is in shock.

7. List at least three intervention techniques for the management
    of seizures.

8. Identify at least five signs of a possible myocardial infarction.

9. Describe the intervention techniques for a person experiencing
    chest pain.

10. List the two guidelines to be followed for all unconscious patients.

11. Name and describe the four kinds of burns and the interventions
    for each.

12. Describe the three common signs for both a fracture and a sprain
    and the appropriate intervention techniques for each.

Key Terms

- anticoagulant
- antidote
- cardiac arrest
- cardiac compressions
- emetic
- finger sweep
- head-tilt/chin-lift maneuver
- Heimlich maneuver
- hypovolemic shock
- jaw-thrust maneuver

- log roll
- Medic-Alert
- Poison Control
- primary survey
- secondary survey
- seizure
- syncope
- tongue-jaw lift
- toxic

Chapter Overview

Chapter Eighteen of the textbook provides basic information about first aid for common emergencies. Working in a hospital does not preclude a healthcare worker from encountering several types of emergencies. Although the hospital environment is considered a *controlled environment*, remember that the patient's health conditions and responses to interventions are often *uncontrolled*.

Review and practice the skills contained in this chapter. Remember the anatomy and physiology from the previous chapters and put it all together. Use the appropriate patient care equipment to practice your skills and learn, learn, learn!

Reading Assignment

Read pages 18-1 through 18-42.

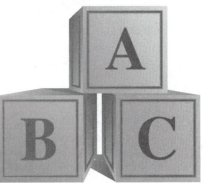

Remember the ABCs of the primary survey: airway, breathing, and circulation.

Name _____

Date _____

Student Enrichment Activities

Complete the following statements.

1. _____ _____ is the immediate care provided to a person who has sustained an unexpected injury, sudden illness, or other medical emergency.

2. The _____ _____ involves assessing the patient for any life-threatening emergencies.

3. The primary survey should be completed in _____ _____ or less.

4. The three parts of the primary survey are: A for _____, B for _____, and C for _____.

5. The two recommended ways of opening an airway are the _____ _____ and the _____ _____.

6. _____ _____ is the method that should be applied first when attempting to control bleeding.

7. Reassessment of the patient is called the _____ _____.

8. Severe shock due to extreme blood loss is called _____ shock.

9. Two causes of seizures are _____ and _____ _____.

10. List four warning signs of a possible myocardial infarction.

    A. _____

    B. _____

    C. _____

    D. _____

11. List three respiratory diseases: _____,

    _____, and _____.

12. Sudden, brief, and temporary loss of consciousness is called _____.

13. Four possible warning signs of impending syncope include:

    A. _____   C. _____

    B. _____   D. _____

14. Poisonings can be _____, or they can be

    _____.

15. An oral emetic used for poisoning is _____ _____ _____.

16. List the four types of burns:

    A. _____   C. _____

    B. _____   D. _____

17. A _____ is an injury to ligaments and tendons.

18. Patients who have hypertension may experience spontaneous

    _____.

Name _____

Date _____

Unscramble the following terms.

19. NOSIPO CTNOOLR   _____   _____

20. CRADICA STARRE   _____   _____

21. SRIFT AID   _____   _____

22. SNOBARIA   _____

23. GLO ORLL   _____   _____

24. SLAUVION   _____

25. ZIERUSE   _____

26. XIOCT   _____

27. SCOPENY   _____

28. SCRIESON   _____

29. MYPLHVOOEIC SCKHO   _____   _____

30. SHOCCIMESY   _____

Name _____

Date _____

Additional Enrichment Activities

Circle the correct answer.

31. If rescue breathing is performed on an adult, delivery of a breath occurs at the rate of:

    A. 1 breath every 4 seconds.

    B. 1 breath every 3 seconds.

    C. 1 breath every 5 seconds.

    D. 2 breaths initially, then 1 breath every 6 seconds.

32. The compression to ventilation ratio during CPR for an infant is:

    A. 2:5.

    B. 5:2.

    C. 1:5.

    D. 5:1.

33. The rate of compressions delivered to an adult during CPR is:

    A. 80 to 100 per minute.

    B. 60 to 80 per minute.

    C. 60 to 100 per minute.

    D. at least 100 per minute.

34. Child and infant rescue breathing is delivered at which rate?

    A. 1 breath every 4 seconds

    B. 1 breath every 3 seconds

    C. 1 breath every 5 seconds

    D. 2 breaths initially, then 1 breath every 4 seconds

35. Management of a foreign body airway obstruction for an infant includes all of the following EXCEPT:

    A. abdominal thrusts can be used if done carefully.

    B. the finger sweep is used if the object is first visualized.

    C. chest thrusts are alternated with back blows.

    D. fingertip placement is the same as that used for chest compressions.

36. When performing a log roll, the person in charge is located:

    A. at the patient's shoulders.

    B. at the patient's hips.

    C. at the patient's head.

    D. at the patient's feet.

37. A common injury that occurs to tendons and ligaments is a:

    A. strain.

    B. sprain.

    C. fracture.

    D. dislocation.

38. The first step in the management of epistaxis is to:

    A. pinch the nostrils.

    B. apply cold packs to nose.

    C. suction the nares.

    D. have the patient sit up if no neck injury is suspected.

39. Injection of a poison may occur:

    A. through insect or arthropod bites.

    B. through reptile bites.

    C. needles.

    D. all of the above.

Name _____

Date _____

40. In the event of poisoning, an oral emetic that is commonly used is:

   A. imodium.

   B. syrup of ipecac.

   C. mustard mixed in salt water.

   D. liquid charcoal.

41. The most common age group in which accidental poisonings occur is:

   A. individuals over 65, due to kidney failure.

   B. adolescents from 13 to 18 years old.

   C. children from 1 to 5 years old.

   D. individuals from 35 to 45 years old.

42. Chemical burns should be flushed for at least:

   A. 20 minutes.

   B. 10 minutes.

   C. 60 minutes.

   D. 5 minutes.

43. Syncope is defined as:

   A. shortness of breath, dyspnea.

   B. seizures.

   C. chaotic firing of neurons within the brain.

   D. sudden, brief, and temporary loss of consciousness.

44. The appropriate pressure point to control bleeding in the leg is on the:

   A. brachial artery.

   B. ulnar artery.

   C. subclavian artery.

   D. femoral artery.

45. The main objective of the primary survey is to:
    A. provide a complete head-to-toe exam for injuries.
    B. survey the scene for any hazards.
    C. detect and correct any life- or limb-threatening emergencies.
    D. notify the appropriate personnel of the situation.

46. The main objective of the secondary survey is to:
    A. provide a complete head-to-toe exam for injuries.
    B. survey the scene for any hazards.
    C. detect and correct any life- or limb-threatening emergencies.
    D. notify the appropriate personnel of the situation.

47. When performing compressions on an adult, the chest should be compressed:
    A. 1- $1^1/_2$ inches.
    B. $2^1/_2$ - 3 inches.
    C. $1^1/_2$ - 2 inches.
    D. 2 - $2^1/_2$ inches.

48. An infant's chest should be compressed _____ when performing chest compressions.
    A. not deeper than $^1/_2$ inch
    B. $1^1/_2$ - 2 inches
    C. 1 - $1^1/_2$ inches
    D. $^1/_2$ - 1 inch

49. Compressions usually are performed on a child using:
    A. the heel of one hand.
    B. the fingertips of one hand and the other hand holding the wrist of that hand.
    C. both hands.
    D. an automatic compression device.

Name _____

Date _____

50. When a person has a partial airway obstruction, they are able to:

    A. cough.

    B. speak.

    C. whisper.

    D. all of the above.

Complete the following exercises.

51. Describe the steps for relieving a foreign body airway obstruction in a CONSCIOUS adult.

_____

_____

_____

_____

_____

_____

52. Describe the steps for performing CPR on a child and infant.

_____

_____

_____

_____

_____

_____

_____

_____

_____

_____

_____

_____

Match the terms in Column A with the appropriate description in Column B.

Column A

53. _____ partial thickness

54. _____ Heimlich maneuver

55. _____ Syrup of Ipecac

56. _____ Log roll

57. _____ hemorrhage

58. _____ antidote

59. _____ at least 80

60. _____ look, listen, and feel

61. _____ tongue-jaw lift

62. _____ adult rescue breathing

63. _____ sniffing position

64. _____ primary survey

65. _____ 5:1

66. _____ 15:2

67. _____ seizure

Column B

A. 1 breath every 5 seconds

B. how to determine breathlessness

C. the ratio of compressions to breaths for adult CPR

D. the proper procedure for turning a patient when spinal injury is suspected or confirmed

E. a method used to detect and correct life and/or limb-threatening emergencies

F. a method of opening the mouth in order to perform a finger sweep

G. describes an extremely painful burn in which damage extends through the epidermis and into the dermis

H. the number of compressions to be completed in 1 minute of adult CPR

I. a procedure used to relieve a foreign body airway obstruction

J. the severe, abnormal internal or external discharge of blood

K. the ratio of compressions to ventilations during infant CPR

L. a neurological dysfunction caused by a sudden episode of uncontrolled electrical activity in the brain

M. an oral emetic

N. a substance that neutralizes a poison

O. the position for opening the airway on an infant

Name _____

Date _____

68. Describe the steps, in order of priority, for controlling active bleeding.

_____

_____

_____

_____

_____

69. Describe the appearance of the following burns.

A. superficial burn: _____

_____

B. partial thickness burn: _____

_____

C. full thickness burn: _____

_____

70. Describe the steps for performing adult CPR.

_____

_____

_____

_____

_____

_____

_____

_____

_____

71. Describe the three methods of opening an airway.

_____

_____

_____

_____

_____

_____

_____

72. Explain the rationale for performing a log roll and provide one example of when you would consider its use.

_____

_____

_____

_____

_____

_____

_____

73. Explain the four ways toxic substances could enter the body.

_____

_____

_____

_____

_____

Name _____

Date _____

74. Name the Methods for Opening an Airway

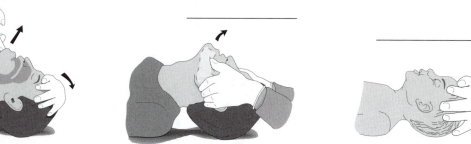

Fill in the blanks for each of the following diagrams.

75. Rescue Breathing

Rescue Breathing		
Adult	_____ breath every _____ seconds	
Child	_____ breath every _____ seconds	
Infant	_____ breath every _____ seconds	

76. CPR

CPR	INFANT ONE PERSON	CHILD (1 - 8 yrs) ONE PERSON	TWO PERSON	ADULT (over 8 yrs) ONE PERSON	TWO PERSON
INITIAL BREATHS					
COMPRESSIONS to BREATHS					
COMPRESSIONS PER MINUTE					
COMPRESS THE STERNUM					
APPLICATIONS					

77. Indirect Pressure Points

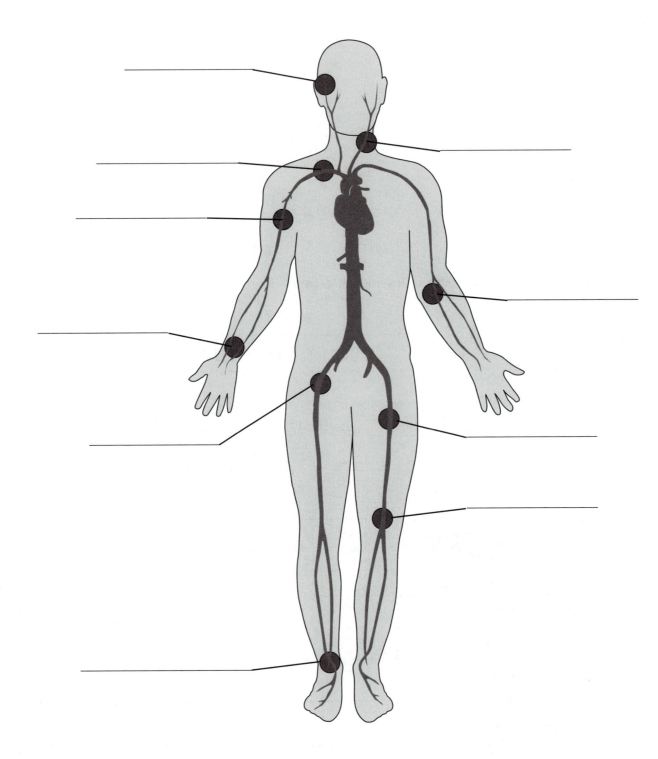

Name _____

Date _____

78. Levels of Burns According to Tissue Layer Damage

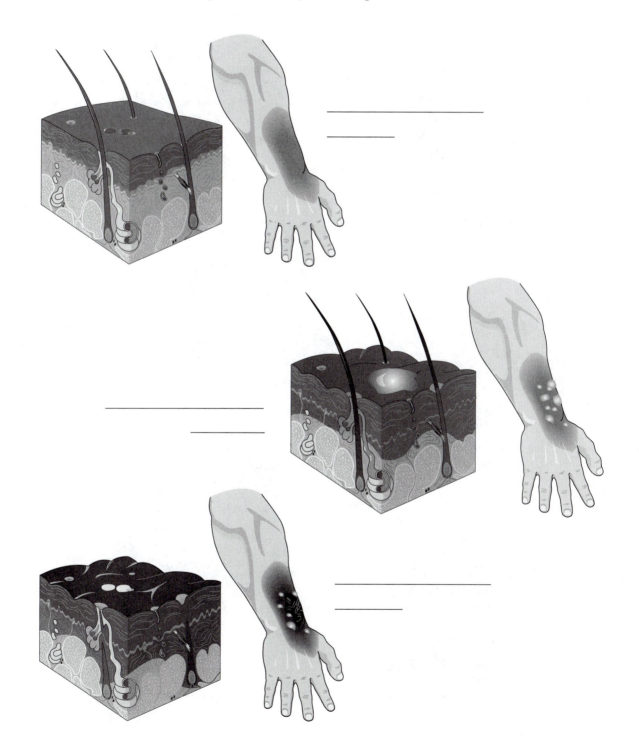

_____

_____

_____

_____

_____

_____

79. Types of Wounds

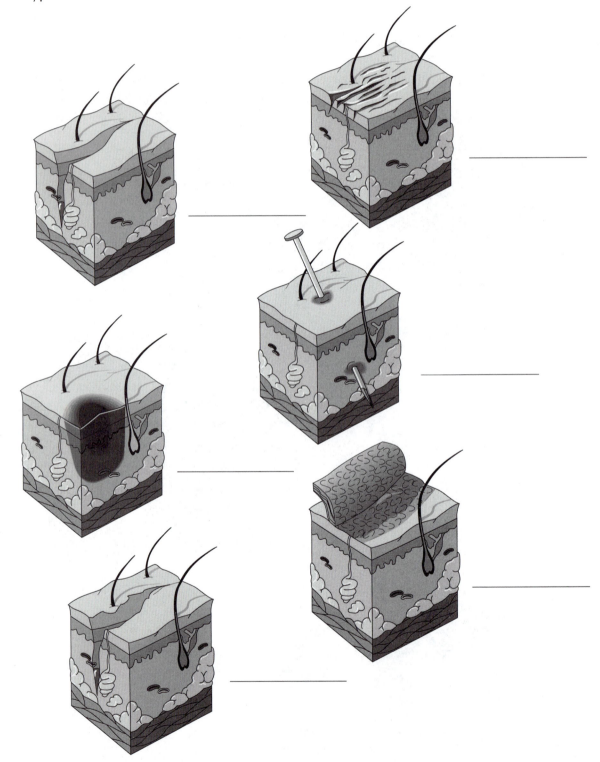

Name _____

Date _____

Basic First Aid—Puzzle 1

Across

3. See 6 Down
4. An injury to soft tissue in which a flap of tissue is torn loose or pulled off
10. An injury to the soft tissues of a joint, characterized by pain, deformity, and the inability to move
12. Describes a patient who is perspiring profusely
14. A maneuver for opening a blocked airway (4 words)
17. Drawing in by suction

Down

1. Fainting; sudden, brief loss of consciousness
2. The black and blue color caused by seepage of blood into tissue as in a contusion
5. A neurological dysfunction that may result in involuntary, uncontrolled muscle contractions
6. A heart attack; a condition caused by the blockage of one or more coronary arteries; with 3 Across

7. The absence of a heartbeat (2 words)
8. An emetic used to induce vomiting (3 words)
9. The immediate care provided to a person involved in a medical emergency (2 words)
11. Tissue death caused by a lack of oxygen
13. A maneuver used to open the airway in a neck-injured patient (2 words)
15. Poisonous
16. Method used to turn a patient with suspected spinal injury (2 words)

Name _____

Date _____

Basic First Aid—Puzzle 2

Find the listed words in the puzzle and circle them. (Contains backwards words.)

E	C	C	H	Y	M	O	S	I	S	O	Z	N	S	C	T	A	N	D	Z
E	P	I	S	T	A	X	I	S	P	T	C	F	G	W	L	E	R	F	T
F	Z	M	L	P	R	D	V	P	Y	T	S	U	R	H	T	W	A	J	S
H	A	T	K	E	Q	A	H	J	Z	A	P	E	Y	J	G	J	J	E	P
F	N	D	X	K	J	Z	P	P	D	Z	D	Y	I	T	Q	V	I	S	Q
S	R	L	N	V	E	X	U	O	F	E	Q	I	O	F	B	Z	I	N	A
K	Y	A	E	M	Y	C	K	Y	Q	L	R	C	D	G	U	S	O	B	C
K	A	N	C	T	E	J	D	D	Z	W	T	Y	U	R	O	I	R	A	T
P	T	E	C	T	O	D	Q	K	O	W	G	X	E	R	S	A	R	K	Z
D	Z	G	V	O	U	D	I	K	X	L	N	P	C	L	S	D	B	Y	B
C	H	H	C	U	P	R	I	C	E	M	U	E	U	I	I	O	B	D	W
F	R	V	Z	C	T	E	E	T	A	Y	N	V	O	A	K	E	S	L	Y
B	P	W	U	W	S	T	C	L	N	L	A	N	C	V	U	Y	M	H	V
G	H	S	X	Z	S	O	L	T	O	A	E	A	E	T	M	J	A	E	R
E	L	K	S	P	G	O	R	K	M	G	R	R	S	X	Z	J	G	G	O
K	R	G	C	N	C	I	R	J	T	R	R	F	T	J	P	S	H	H	M
K	S	A	A	L	Q	F	D	O	E	V	J	O	N	T	E	O	B	K	H
K	X	R	K	H	P	P	X	S	Q	B	H	Y	L	A	A	I	G	V	J
C	G	J	B	K	V	I	T	R	F	S	I	N	Q	L	J	G	L	I	V
K	A	N	A	I	C	Z	D	M	V	V	Y	V	A	B	C	Z	F	T	R

ABRASION	JAW THRUST
ANTIDOTE	LOG ROLL
AVULSION	MEDIC ALERT TAG
CARDIAC ARREST	NECROSIS
ECCHYMOSIS	SEIZURE
EPISTAXIS	SYNCOPE
FRACTURE	TOXIC

Chapter Nineteen
Healthful Living

Objectives

After completing this chapter you should be able to
do the following:

1. Define and correctly spell each of the key terms.

2. Describe the concept of preventive healthcare.

3. Identify the health risks associated with the inhalation of
    tobacco smoke.

4. Identify the difference between essential and secondary
    hypertension.

5. Describe the health risks associated with untreated hypertension.

6. Identify measures for maintaining ideal blood pressure.

7. List the health problems often seen in patients who chronically
    abuse alcohol and drugs.

8. Understand the concepts of stress and coping mechanisms.

9. Identify the nutritional and energy values of carbohydrates, fats,
    and proteins.

10. Explain the function of each type of cholesterol carrier.

11. Identify health risks for those who are overweight.

Key Terms

- aerobic
- basal metabolic rate
- calorie
- carbohydrate
- cholesterol
- fat

- high-density lipoprotein
- low-density lipoprotein
- minerals
- preventive healthcare
- protein
- vitamins

Chapter Overview

As a healthcare worker, you must learn to fill the role of a patient educator. Chapter Nineteen discusses factors that are known to cause stress, coping mechanisms that can be used to manage stress, and habits that are harmful to one's health.

This information is not only important to patients, but also to those who work in healthcare. Keeping yourself healthy allows you to better care for your patients. Maintaining a healthy outlook also sets an example for your patients, family, and friends to follow. Use the information contained in this chapter to better educate the general public and to become the best role model for patients. Everyone's health is important.

Reading Assignment

Read pages 19-1 through 19-19.

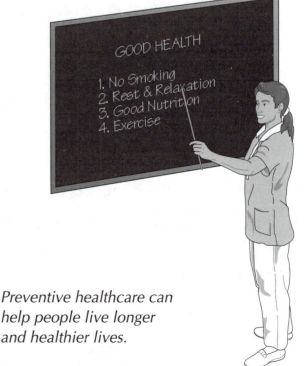

Preventive healthcare can help people live longer and healthier lives.

Name _____

Date _____

Student Enrichment Activities

Complete the following statements.

1. A substance that causes cancer is called a _____.

2. A toxic substance that is found in all parts of the tobacco plant is _____.

3. Hypertension without an apparent medical cause is _____
   _____.

4. One's _____ _____ often determine whether stress will be positive or negative.

5. Five ways to effectively manage stress include the following:
   A. _____   D. _____
   B. _____   E. _____
   C. _____

6. A healthy diet should be made up of _____ % carbohydrates, _____ % fats, and _____ % protein.

7. The principal source of energy for the body is provided by _____.

8. Carbohydrates are broken down into _____.

9. Fats are needed in order to transport vitamins _____, _____, _____, and _____.

10. The primary building block of any body part is _____.

11. A waxy, white substance made from fat is _____.

12. Cholesterol-carriers contained in the body are _____.

13. The rate at which the body normally burns calories is the _____ _____ _____.

Unscramble the following terms.

14. ASALB CIMETBOLA TERA   _____ _____ _____

15. YGLONCEG   _____

16. TINCIONE   _____

17. SLENTI KRELLI   _____ _____

18. WALWITHARD   _____

19. SSSTER   _____

20. TRIPONE   _____

21. TRIOPLEPION   _____

22. GARCIONCEN   _____

23. EROACIL   _____

24. BROAICE   _____

Name _____

Date _____

Additional Enrichment Activities

Circle the correct answer.

25. Cholesterol is made from:

    A. carbohydrates.

    B. fats.

    C. roughage.

    D. vegetarian foods.

26. The most efficient method of burning fat calories is:

    A. anaerobic exercise.

    B. living a sedentary lifestyle.

    C. aerobic exercise.

    D. drinking over 64 ounces of water daily.

27. The basal metabolic rate is controlled and determined by the:

    A. thyroid gland.

    B. pituitary gland.

    C. sex glands.

    D. parathyroid glands.

28. The risk of cancer increases by _____ times if two packs of cigarettes per day are smoked, or if one has smoked for twenty years.

    A. 50

    B. 100

    C. 20

    D. 25

29. Nicotine is classified as a (an):
    A. analgesic.
    B. carcinogen.
    C. anesthetic.
    D. all of the above.

30. An alcohol-dependent patient who is hospitalized will usually manifest withdrawal symptoms within:
    A. 24 to 48 hrs.
    B. 48 to 72 hrs.
    C. 12 to 36 hrs.
    D. 72 to 96 hrs.

31. The principal sources of energy for the body are:
    A. proteins.
    B. fats.
    C. carbohydrates.
    D. vitamins.

32. The percentage of total caloric intake from fats should not exceed:
    A. 30%.
    B. 55%.
    C. 15%.
    D. 25%.

33. The primary building blocks of all body parts are:
    A. vitamins.
    B. fats.
    C. proteins.
    D. carbohydrates.

Name _____

Date _____

34. The type of cholesterol carriers that remove some of the cholesterol from the blood are:

    A. HDLs.

    B. LDLs.

    C. DLHs.

    D. none of the above.

Complete the following exercises.

35. Due to the systemic effects of nicotine and the central effects of cigarette smoke on the lungs, patients with which diseases should especially be discouraged from smoking?

    _____

    _____

    _____

    _____

    _____

    _____

36. Discuss the role of lipoproteins in the body's management of cholesterol.

    _____

    _____

    _____

    _____

    _____

    _____

    _____

37. Define the following terms.

    A. essential hypertension:_____

    _____

    B. secondary hypertension: _____

    _____

38. Define and discuss each of the following terms.

    A. fat: _____

    _____

    _____

    _____

    B. carbohydrate: _____

    _____

    _____

    _____

    C. protein: _____

    _____

    _____

    _____

    D. vitamins: _____

    _____

    _____

    _____

    E. minerals:_____

    _____

    _____

    _____

Name _____

Date _____

Healthful Living—Puzzle 1

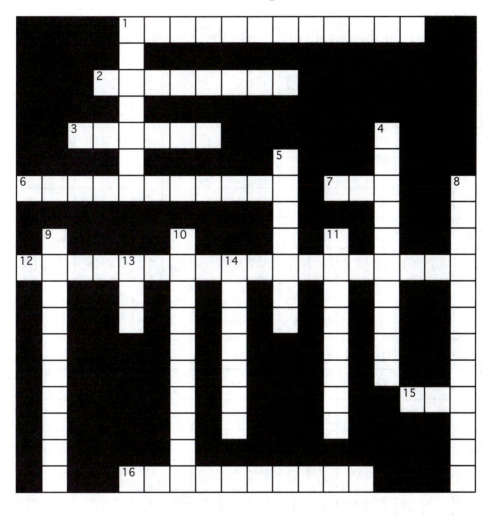

Across

1. A complex sugar that is a basic source of energy
2. A carbohydrate made of glucose that is stored in the liver and muscles
3. A perceived challenge to one's coping mechanisms
6. A waxy, white substance made from fat
7. A source of energy made up of lipids or fatty acids
12. The rate at which the body burns calories while at rest
15. Abbreviation for high density lipoprotein
16. Focuses on patient education that emphasizes promotion of health and prevention of disease; with 10 Down

Down

1. A measure of a unit of heat
4. Symptoms that occur after quitting drugs or alcohol
5. A simple sugar used in the human body
8. A descriptive term for hypertension
9. A cancer-causing substance
10. See 16 Across
11. An addictive poison found in tobacco plants
13. Abbreviation for low density lipoprotein
14. Requires oxygen

Name _____

Date _____

Healthful Living—Puzzle 2

Find the listed words in the puzzle and circle them. (Contains backwards words.)

L	I	P	O	P	R	O	T	E	I	N	S	H	C	L	L
S	I	L	E	N	T	K	I	L	L	E	R	W	U	H	G
C	R	J	U	W	Z	K	C	Z	K	M	J	X	E	L	W
E	A	U	F	U	J	K	K	G	Q	G	R	S	Y	C	I
P	I	R	E	I	I	T	Q	K	X	S	O	C	O	I	T
Z	R	R	B	D	Z	S	C	Q	S	C	O	M	L	O	H
N	G	O	O	V	O	N	M	U	G	P	O	P	J	D
F	J	D	T	L	H	M	G	L	E	L	J	F	T	K	R
V	B	P	E	E	A	Y	G	N	E	U	Z	A	Y	K	A
V	J	Y	B	M	I	C	D	X	K	N	L	T	Y	M	W
W	Y	C	R	J	S	N	S	R	I	L	N	T	K	E	A
H	I	S	P	T	G	U	S	F	A	F	P	B	E	H	L
S	E	N	R	K	G	S	I	G	A	T	T	F	H	M	G
E	U	E	J	A	Z	U	X	E	O	T	E	B	D	Y	K
G	S	M	R	M	F	I	Z	M	F	R	S	S	D	J	B
S	C	A	R	C	I	N	O	G	E	N	Z	X	P	D	K

CALORIE	GLYCOGEN
CARBOHYDRATES	LIPOPROTEINS
CARCINOGEN	PROTEIN
COMPLEX SUGAR	SILENT KILLER
FATS	STRESS
GLUCOSE	WITHDRAWAL

Chapter Twenty
Career Planning

Objectives

After completing this chapter you should be able to
do the following:

1. Define and correctly spell each of the key terms.

2. Identify and describe at least four resources for locating
    job openings.

3. Explain the difference between a job and a career.

4. Identify at least five areas to evaluate during a self-assessment
    prior to writing your resumé.

5. Write your resumé.

6. Write a cover letter.

7. Identify at least six guidelines to consider when preparing for
    an interview.

8. Identify the four aspects of being a positive influence on the
    healthcare team.

9. List the Ten Commandments of Human Relations.

Key Terms

- career
- cover letter

- job
- resumé

Chapter Overview

Chapter Twenty marks the end of an intensive introductory course in clinical allied healthcare. You have worked hard to reach this point in your education, and now it is time to start the hunt for a position in which you can put your training to use.

This chapter describes the skills you will need to begin your career: how to find an entry-level position, how to assess your personal attributes, how to write cover letters and resumés, and how to make a good impression during your employment interview. Practice these skills by actively participating in role-playing exercises. It is important to polish your skills before you enter the *real world*. After all, first impressions are lasting impressions!

Reading Assignment

Read pages 20-1 through 20-18.

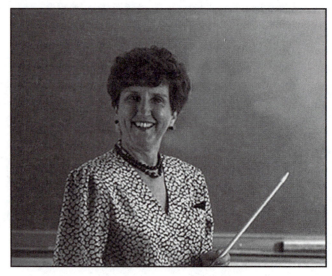

Your instructor may be a good source of information regarding potential positions.

Name _____

Date _____

Student Enrichment Activities

1. Resources available to assist in finding an entry-level position include

   _____, _____, _____,

   _____, and _____.

2. Aspects of proper telephone etiquette include _____,

   _____, _____, and _____.

3. Identify seven areas of self-assessment that all job applicants should honestly evaluate:

   A. _____   **E.** _____

   B. _____   **F.** _____

   C. _____   **G.** _____

   D. _____

4. In addition to the heading, the categories that are generally included on all resumés

   are the _____ _____, the _____ _____

   _____, and the _____ _____.

5. List seven questions that are commonly asked of job applicants during an interview.

   A. _____

   B. _____

   C. _____

   D. _____

   E. _____

   F. _____

   G. _____

6. Write your resumé and a cover letter. Role play in small groups by reviewing each other's documents and assist each other in *polishing* them up.

Name _____

Date _____

Additional Enrichment Activities

Circle the correct answer.

7. A career:

   A. is one's lifelong work.

   B. often allows one to achieve self-actualization.

   C. often involves steady progression.

   D. all of the above.

8. Information regarding career positions may be obtained:

   A. by networking.

   B. from your instructor or instructors.

   C. from newspaper advertisements.

   D. all of the above.

9. When writing your resumé, do all of the following EXCEPT:

   A. use a word processor.

   B. use common terminology and phrases.

   C. use white out to cover errors.

   D. limit the length of the resumé.

10. It is acceptable to omit high school education information on a resumé if you have been out of school:

    A. over five years.

    B. high school education must always be included.

    C. over ten years.

    D. over twenty years.

11. During the interview:

    A. maintain good eye contact.

    B. wear fashionable clothes.

    C. take a friend for support and encouragement.

    D. do not ask questions of the interviewer.

Complete the following exercises.

12. List and explain each of the Ten Commandments of Human Relations.

_____

_____

_____

_____

_____

_____

_____

_____

_____

_____

_____

_____

_____

_____

_____

13. List four attitudes of the *ideal employee.*

_____

_____

_____

Name _____

Date _____

14. Describe the organization of a resumé.

_____

_____

_____

_____

_____

_____

15. List and describe at least five sources that may provide information on healthcare-oriented positions.

_____

_____

_____

_____

_____

_____

_____

_____

_____

_____

16. Itemize eight guidelines that can help you give a good first impression on the telephone.

_____

_____

_____

_____

_____

_____

_____

_____

17. List the seven qualities for which an employer may look that require self-assessment before writing a resumé.

_____

_____

_____

_____

_____

_____

Name _____

Date _____

Career Planning—Puzzle 1

Across

4. Verbal or nonverbal exchange of messages, thoughts, ideas, and feelings
5. The drive to first begin an action
6. A profession for which one trains and that is undertaken as one's lifelong work
8. Related to past experience, knowledge, or education
10. Characteristics which make a person fit for a job
12. A piece of writing that accompanies a resume to explain or introduce its contents (2 words)
13. The way one looks, including clothes, grooming habits, facial expressions
14. The number of times a person is present or available to perform certain obligations, as at work

Down

1. The degree of reliance or trust that can be placed in a person
2. A specific role that is performed regularly for compensation
3. Working together in a harmonious fashion to accomplish a goal
7. A brief, written account of personal and professional qualifications and experience
9. Something desired and for which an effort is made
11. Honesty

Name _____

Date _____

Career Planning—Puzzle 2

Find the listed words in the puzzle and circle them. (Contains backwards words.)

O	Q	D	E	N	A	A	M	Z	L	F	M	U	D	Z	T	H	C	W	Z
K	N	M	O	F	Y	Y	T	I	C	V	S	R	B	Z	B	L	X	R	B
T	Q	C	M	M	X	T	C	T	R	Z	X	C	F	V	B	I	W	V	N
O	I	G	O	V	N	Y	I	C	E	E	U	K	N	E	X	R	E	F	I
E	D	F	A	U	Q	T	P	L	O	N	F	S	W	H	R	Z	R	E	M
R	X	W	M	P	T	T	A	Z	I	V	D	E	Y	H	V	X	B	Z	C
B	L	C	V	Z	W	Z	K	Z	N	B	E	A	R	G	M	K	F	A	Z
M	X	D	F	N	S	P	S	G	Y	C	A	R	N	E	H	H	C	Y	W
P	W	S	J	Q	Z	P	B	P	O	W	I	D	L	C	N	A	P	O	E
K	B	X	F	P	K	B	Z	O	E	N	I	G	N	E	E	C	X	Y	Y
G	F	Y	K	K	Q	N	P	C	I	N	J	E	R	E	T	R	E	V	O
U	Y	Z	F	N	U	E	N	T	T	B	D	S	E	Z	P	T	X	S	Q
D	W	S	Y	K	R	A	I	E	V	P	Z	G	H	Z	S	E	E	E	G
D	F	H	A	A	R	A	G	P	S	B	E	X	V	I	Y	V	D	R	T
S	L	M	T	A	T	R	E	Z	R	C	A	E	S	D	Y	M	L	Y	Z
T	P	I	E	I	I	Q	E	N	O	J	Y	B	M	L	Q	I	N	X	B
G	O	P	V	T	U	E	K	R	Q	O	G	D	D	D	W	R	W	D	O
N	P	E	Y	V	L	J	C	V	S	Y	L	M	P	K	Z	G	G	I	J
A	W	F	O	F	X	V	X	P	C	K	A	O	P	E	M	U	S	E	R
Y	S	X	U	T	W	N	U	R	L	I	V	D	R	R	E	E	R	A	C

APPEARANCE

ATTENDANCE

CAREER

COOPERATION

COVER LETTER

DEPENDABILITY

INITIATIVE

INTEGRITY

JOB

REFERENCES

RESUME